The Eight-Step Approach to Teaching Clinical Nursing

The Eight-Step Approach to Teaching Clinical Nursing

TOOLS FOR NURSE EDUCATORS

JoAnne Herman, PhD, RN
Assistant Dean for Graduate
    Studies
Associate Professor
College of Nursing,
University of South Carolina
Columbia, South Carolina

Loretta Manning, MSN, RN, GNP
President
I CAN Publishing®, Inc.
Educational Consultant
Duluth, Georgia

Lydia R. Zager, MSN, RN
Clinical Professor
Medical/Surgical Nursing
    Coordinator,
College of Nursing,
University of South Carolina
Columbia, South Carolina

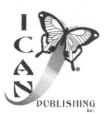

I CAN Publishing®, Inc. ◆ Duluth, GA
www.icanpublishing.com

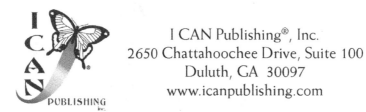

I CAN Publishing®, Inc.
2650 Chattahoochee Drive, Suite 100
Duluth, GA 30097
www.icanpublishing.com

The publisher is dedicated to provide competent and reliable information regarding the subject matter covered. However, it is sold with the understanding that the authors and publisher are not engaged in rendering legal or other professional advice. Nurse Practice Acts often vary from state to state and if legal or other expert assistance is required, the services of a professional should be sought. The authors and publisher specifically disclaim any liability that is incurred from the use or application of the contents of this book.

ISBN: 978-0-9842040-4-5
Library of Congress Control Number: 2010943147
Printed in the United States of America
First Edition

Copies of this book may be obtained from:
I CAN Publishing®, Inc.
2650 Chattahoochee Drive, Suite 100
Duluth, GA 30097
1-866-428-5589
www.icanpublishing.com

Cover and interior design by Mary Jo Zazueta/www.tothepointsolutions.com

Contents

About the Authors

DR. JOANNE HERMAN received her PhD in nursing from the University of Texas at Austin. One of her major scholarship activities has been clinical reasoning. She provided leadership in a curriculum revision at the University of South Carolina College of Nursing in 1985 that resulted in the addition of two courses in clinical reasoning. She taught the senior level baccalaureate course for 10 years. In 1995, the curriculum was revised again and she taught the junior level clinical reasoning course. JoAnne was awarded the prestigious Michael. J. Mungo award for undergraduate teaching at the University of South Carolina. She is a known national and international speaker and has been a frequent presenter at many nursing conferences. She is the co-author of *Clinical Reasoning: The Art and Science of Critical and Creative Thinking*. She has multiple publications both theoretical and clinical application related to clinical reasoning. She has served as a consultant for soft ware companies who wanted to include clinical reasoning as the basis for their content presentations.

LORETTA S. MANNING received her MSN from Indiana University and her BSN from Indiana State University. She received her Gerontological Nurse Practitioner certificate from the University of North Carolina in Greensboro, North Carolina. After working as an intensive critical care and charge nurse in pediatric nursing, she became a clinical educator at the University of Indianapolis. In 1984, she taught in the BSN program at Northwestern State University, in Shreveport, Louisiana. Loretta has co-authored *Nursing Made Insanely Easy, Pharmacology Made Insanely Easy, NCLEX-RN® 101: How to Pass*, and *Pathways of Teaching Nursing: Keeping it Real*. Loretta is a 2004 graduate fellow of the Amy V. Cockcroft Leadership Development Program. She has consulted with schools nationally and internationally in assisting faculty with teaching strategies, for making learning fun and assisting with clinical decision making. Loretta's expertise is in developing faculty and clinical adjunct instructors in the area of connecting NCLEX®, Patient Safety, and Joint Commission Standards both in the classroom as well as in clinical education. She has one chapter on preparing students for the NCLEX-RN® published in 2008 in the book, *Mastering the Teaching Role: A Guide for Nurse Educators*. She has recently co-developed a medical surgical concept curriculum. Loretta Manning is the President and Co-Founder of I CAN Publishing®, Inc., a company dedicated to improving health care and inspiring educators and learners by transforming education through creating resources to make teaching and learning easy and fun.

LYDIA R. ZAGER earned her MSN in nursing administration with a minor in education at the University of Texas in San Antonio, Texas and her BSN from Pittsburg State University in Pittsburg, Kansas. She is currently a clinical professor in the College of Nursing at the University of South Carolina since 1998. Prior to that, she was a clinical faculty for Central Carolina Technical

College. Lydia is a retired Lieutenant Colonel from the Army Nurse Corps and served in a variety of leadership positions in the military to include clinical management, staff advisor, recruitment and chief of hospital education. Lydia is a 2004 graduate fellow of the Amy V. Cockcroft Leadership Development Program. Lydia has gained national and state recognition in clinical nursing education through her consulting, presentations and faculty development workshops. Her expertise is in developing clinical and adjunct nursing instructors particularly in the area of clinical reasoning and organizing the clinical day to help meet patient safety, NCLEX® and Joint Commission Standards. In addition she has years of experience in teaching preceptor workshops and facilitating preceptor programs. She has two chapters on leadership and the multigenerational student published in 2008 in the book, *Mastering the Teaching Role: A Guide for Nurse Educator* and is the co-author of two articles on leadership. She has recently co-developed a medical surgical concept curriculum.

Preface

"The most important thing in nursing is not so much to gain more and more facts as to TRANSFORM the way we think about these facts."

~ Loretta Manning, President, I CAN Publishing®, Inc.

Effective clinical education is imperative for the success of nursing education programs, student success as well as outcomes for quality patient care. Nursing programs are expected to develop proficient clinicians upon graduation. This mandates that nursing programs provide excellent clinical experiences where students learn to integrate the theory with competent clinical skills in the care of clients.

During our consultations with nursing faculty, we were routinely requested to provide a document including all of the clinical teaching tools that were discussed and reviewed. Faculty requested these tools to assist nursing students in linking theory with clinical decision-making to facilitate both clinical and exam success. They have also requested these tools to simplify the planning and evaluating process during clinical rotations with their students.

We began the journey to write this book because of the numerous requests from clinical faculty. We realized this book needed to have a practical approach to clinical teaching. We want to provide you with the tools and strategies of how to begin teaching clinical nursing day one and proceed to the last day and final clinical evaluations. Rarely do nursing instructors get any formal preparation in the area of clinical education. In the past, becoming an effective clinical instructor was like becoming an effective parent. There was no road map or compass to guide us through the maze. This challenge has multiplied because of the need for numerous part-time clinical instructors. New clinical faculty are often expert clinicians but may have little teaching experience. Since clinical instructors play the pivotal role in connecting theory to practice, it is imperative to assist them in their vital role to maximize student learning in clinical.

This book contains many tools and forms that can be used as templates in clinical. The tools and information included in this book have been developed from our 38 years of combined clinical experience teaching nursing students in academic settings and nurses in a variety of clinical units from across the country.

We hope this book will be a practical guide for clinical teaching. The book is now in your hands to reach your destination.

The Eight-Step Approach to Teaching Clinical Nursing is illustrated by using the word **CLINICAL** as indicated below:

C   Clinical Teaching: How Do I Start?

L   Learn How to Structure the Clinical Day

I   Improve Critical Thinking and Clinical Judgment

N   Nursing Concept Map

I   Interactive Strategies for Clinical Teaching

C   Collaborating with Multi-Generational Learners

A   Assessment and Evaluation

L   Linking Clinical Experience to NCLEX® Success

There are two ways you can approach this book. Our first recommendation is to read the book in its entirety for continuity of content and a complete picture of the clinical teaching process. Another approach to expedite your learning or for a refresher, you can refer directly to the area where you need assistance. We hope this book will facilitate your transition into your clinical educator role and make this a positive experience if you are a new educator. If you are an experienced nursing clinical instructor, we hope the clinical tools will continue to assist you in guiding student's success both on the NCLEX® and in clinical practice and will be a resource as you mentor new clinical instructors.

We dedicate this work to the many nursing faculty who are busy teaching clinical nursing and are constantly striving for an increased level of excellence as a clinical instructor!

Acknowledgments

We want to acknowledge and express our appreciation to the clinical faculty at the University of South Carolina in Columbia, South Carolina. We appreciate your contributions, your helpful suggestions, the adaptation and use of many of the forms in this book throughout the clinical courses.

We also want to thank the nursing students across the country and from the University of South Carolina for all of the useful feedback that has assisted us throughout the development of the tools and book.

We want to express our appreciation to each of our family members for their never-ending support and love while we developed this book.

We want to thank Jennifer Robinson, our Administrative Director, who supports us with all aspects of writing, publishing, and distributing our books. We most want to thank her for her love and great sense of humor that keeps us smiling and laughing during the moments we are working to meet deadlines!

The Eight-Step Approach to Teaching Clinical Nursing

CHAPTER 1

Clinical Teaching: How Do I Start?

IN THIS CHAPTER YOU WILL:

→ Assess your readiness to be a clinical instructor

→ Discover how your novice students think and learn

→ Explore the characteristics of your novice student learners

---

ASSESS YOUR READINESS TO BE A CLINICAL INSTRUCTOR

As a clinical instructor, you are one of the most important and powerful people in preparing new nurses for the future. Through a collaborative partnership with your students in clinical, you can make learning a positive experience that will set the tone for how students approach client care.

Clinical teaching can be a scary process, but not when you are adequately prepared. Through adequate preparation, clinical teaching is extremely rewarding. This chapter will help you assess your readiness to be a clinical instructor. The **Clinical Instructor Self-Assessment Questionnaire** found at the end of this chapter will help you with this process as you begin your role. If the answer to any of the following questions is "No," the resource column will help you find the information you need.

DISCOVER HOW YOUR NOVICE STUDENTS THINK AND LEARN

The brain is structured in neural-networks. These networks are established through learning and experience, which is why clinical is so important in the development of a new nurse. We used to believe, for example, that how we baked a cake was all located in one part of the brain. Now we know through fMRI imaging that the knowledge about how to bake a cake is stored all over the brain. The knowledge about how to bake the cake is accessed as we develop neural-networks with increasing numbers of inter-connections through our experience in baking a cake. The more times we bake the cake, the more inter-connections are established, and the more expertise we develop. That is why you, as an expert nurse, are able to reach clinical decisions very quickly. You have an almost infinite number of inter-connections with stored knowledge because of your extensive experience. The novice learner, your student, has minimal inter-connections.

Initial learning is temporary. Repetition is critical for students to learn. The neural-networks become better connected through increased repetition. For example, every time a student inserts a foley catheter, the relationship among the steps of the procedure, sterile technique, rationale for the foley, potential complications and needed patient teaching increases the strength of the connection of these parts to each other resulting in an increased competence of the student.

EXPLORE THE CHARACTERISTICS OF YOUR NOVICE STUDENT LEARNERS

+ They make decisions quickly before thinking about all the options that are possible, in other words, they will jump to conclusions.

+ They have difficulty applying classroom content to clinical situations.

+ They are easily overwhelmed by data, i.e., information in the medical record.

+ They have difficulty distinguishing relevant from irrelevant information.

+ They have low tolerance for ambiguity—the students just want you to tell them what to do!!!

+ They may be unwilling to engage in challenging problems.

+ They want to rely heavily on known solutions.

+ They often have a non-systematic approach to clinical problems.

In addition, your novice student learner approaches clinical often in a very apprehensive way. They see clinical as a set of tasks that must be accomplished. Each clinical day is a test of their personal capabilities.

So imagine their stress level!! This is why establishing a positive learning environment for students is so important. These characteristics of the novice learner need to be considered in all aspects of clinical: observing care given, providing feedback, questioning and evaluating student performance. The following chapters provide strategies that you can use to help your novice nursing student progress and give you the tools necessary to be an even better clinical instructor.

CLINICAL FACULTY SELF-ASSESSMENT QUESTIONNAIRE

Self-Assessment Questions	Yes, I Know	No, I Need Help	Resources: Where to Find Help
1. Do I understand the expected student outcomes of this clinical?			Refer to course syllabus and course coordinator.
2. Do I have the knowledge, skills and abilities to assist my students in the types of client care that they will give?			1. Refer to course text books. 2. Get clinical experience with similar types of patients. 3. Work with another experienced instructor.
3. Have I oriented to the clinical setting where I will have students? This information should include: staffing, policies and procedures, and medication protocols, documentation, supply systems, safety or quality assurance concerns.			1. Spend time in the clinical setting prior to bringing students to clinical. 2. Review unit and clinical facilities' policies and procedures. 3. Determine orientation and access requirements needed for medication, documentation and supply systems. 4. Determine what orientation is required for the students per unit protocol. 5. Discuss with the nurse manager the safety and QI concerns. 6. Review appropriate orientation.
4. Do I know what the clinical setting offers as learning opportunities for my students?			1. Meet with coordinator at the clinical site and the unit managers where the students will be. 2. Meet with others at the clinical site as appropriate, i.e., OR, ED.
5. Do I know how to prepare the clinical staff and clients for students?			Refer to Chapter 2
6. Do I know how to prepare students by establishing the expectations and structure for the clinical day? This should include: a. orientation to the unit b. the clinical day routine c. documentation d. administer medications e. written plans for care f. pre and post conference			Read Chapter 2

Handout 1

CLINICAL FACULTY SELF-ASSESSMENT QUESTIONNAIRE (cont'd)

Self-Assessment Questions	Yes, I Know	No, I Need Help	Resources: Where to Find Help
7. Do I know how novice students learn and do I know how to apply teaching strategies appropriately?			Chapter 1, 2, 3
8. Do I know how to use NCLEX® activities to organize my teaching?			Refer to chapter 8
9. Do I know how to ask inquiry and reflections questions?			Refer to Chapter 3
10. Do I know how to use a concept map in clinical?			Refer to Chapter 4
11. Do I know how to help students make clinical judgments through the use of thinking strategies?			Refer to Chapter 3
12. Do I know how to use innovative teaching strategies in clinical?			Refer to Chapter 5
13. Do I know how to give formal and informal feedback to my students?			Refer to Chapter 7
14. Do I know how to do counseling for improvement and for failure to meet clinical requirements?			Refer to Chapter 7
15. Do I know how to evaluate students' clinical performance?			Refer to Chapter 7

CHAPTER 2

Learn How to Structure the Clinical Day

IN THIS CHAPTER YOU WILL LEARN HOW TO:

→ Structure the clinical day

→ Structure medication administration

→ Structure how students organize their clinical data

STRUCTURING THE CLINICAL DAY

Many new clinical instructors feel overwhelmed with how to organize a clinical day. The thought of coordinating eight to ten nursing students with medication administration alone can result in a sleepless night. Our goal is to provide you with tools and structure to assist you in planning and organizing the clinical day.

A step often left out, is preparing the unit staff for the students. Good communication with the staff can make all the difference in the quality of the clinical experience and the relationships among the staff, you, and the students. Share with the staff the course syllabus, student learning objectives, skills the students can perform without you, and skills students can do with the nursing staff. Determine how you will communicate student clinical assignments and what aspects of client care students will be performing. Share this information with the staff while you are orienting to the unit.

The next step is to plan your clinical day. The first chart provides an example of how to structure a typical clinical day. When you are working with novice nursing students, they need structure to decrease their anxiety and optimize their learning experience. The chart **How to Structure a Typical Clinical Day**, found at the end of the chapter, can be adapted to your clinical setting. It may seem like a lot of work, but the time spent in planning will help ensure your success.

STRUCTURING MEDICATION ADMINISTRATION

The second chart found at the end of the chapter is a **Medication Protocol: A Fail Safe Approach**. It is imperative that clinical instructors also provide a structure to help students develop safe medication administration practices. When clinical instructors consistently use a structured process, students develop safe medication administration habits essential to prevent medication errors. The medication protocol not only helps students administer medications safely and efficiently, it helps you feel confident that the students are prepared to give their medications.

In order for the medication protocol to have the maximum effect, all clinical instructors must use it throughout the courses. This prevents students from having to learn a new structure for giving medications with each clinical instructor. This consistency throughout the courses provides repetition and strengthens the safe medication administration habit for the students.

STRUCTURE HOW STUDENTS ORGANIZE THEIR CLINICAL DATA

Students are overwhelmed with how to organize the information they get from report and orders for procedures and medications. Without a structured format, students are disorganized in their thinking, delivery of care, and timeliness. This disorganization makes it difficult for students to document accurately. At the end of the chapter is an example of a **Student Report Sheet** that students can use when receiving report at the beginning of clinical.

Also included at the end of the chapter are an example of a **Typical Day Events** and a description of a **Shift Report Using SBAR Format**. We have found these two handouts to be extremely useful to the students in helping them organize their day and learn how to give an effective and accurate report using SBAR.

The most effective use of all of these tools is to share them with the students prior to clinical. The tools help students understand the expectations for clinical performance, document with accuracy, and most importantly, provide safe and effective care in a timely manner.

HOW TO STRUCTURE A TYPICAL CLINICAL DAY

Time	Student Activity	Instructor Reminders and Notes (The following are examples.)
6:45 AM When you arrive for clinical prior to pre-conference time . . .	Get report (SBAR) from your nurse. Check for: • New orders • New medications • Time of 1st medication • Check if NPO for tests, surgery or procedures. If so, will they get any of their meds, i.e., insulin, antihypertensives?	The goal for clinical faculty prior to the beginning of clinical is to determine: • What student, what client, what skills, what medications are going to require your attention? • How will you prioritize and guide the students in prioritizing their activities? Example: • Prioritize the student's learning needs (i.e., Trach suctioning and does the student have the skill?) • Prioritize assigned client's needs (i.e., acuity, medications times; i.e., 7 AM medication) • Know what diagnostic exams (i.e., are they NPO for cardiac cath?)
Pre-conference	Share clinical concept maps and plans for the day	Assess if the students are prepared: • Do they have their clinical concept map with predicted client's needs and interventions and are they accurate? • Use inquiry questions in your assessment • Schedule student activities that require clinical instructor supervision beginning with early AM medications and scheduled procedures
7:00 – 7:20 AM	See your client for a quick assessment: • Respiratory status, in pain, safety issues, etc. • Check IVs. Make sure they are patent and running at the right rate with the right fluid • Check for any other lines, tubes, that they are patent, and note the drainage • Take B/P and pulse • Check on blood sugars or obtain glucometer reading • Administer insulin or other before meals medications • (Always check to see if the med has been given, is being held, etc.) • Prepare for any scheduled tests	• Use Medication protocol • Meet students as scheduled

HOW TO STRUCTURE A TYPICAL CLINICAL DAY (cont'd)

Time	Student Activity	Instructor Reminders and Notes (The following are examples.)
8:00 – 9:30 AM	• Give AM medications • Perform other client procedures as ordered • Prepare client for scheduled procedures/surgery if scheduled • Complete physical assessment • Complete or ensure AM care is done (often a good time to assess and do your physical)	• Use medication protocol • Divide students into groups • Have part of the students begin with medication administration • Have part of the students complete AM care and do assessments • Recommend doing procedures that require supervision after AM medications are given
9:30 – 10 AM	• First documentation entered to include assessments and other findings • Implement and evaluate your nursing interventions, i.e., coughing and deep breathing • Turn or ambulate your client • Assess activity tolerance	Begin making rounds of student's clients: • See priority clients first, i.e. and indwelling lines, IVs, tubes, unstable clients • Facilitate students with their care • Ask students inquiry questions &/or reflection questions (see chart in Chapter 3 for suggestions)
10:30 AM	• Continue to assess client and document • Evaluate response to PRN medications • Complete any treatments or procedures as ordered (This may be earlier depending on the time of the test) • Client teaching and documentation • Continue to check for new doctor's orders • Check for lab result, i.e., PTT if on heparin	• Ensure students have completed assessments, evaluations and documents of client's progress toward outcomes • Assist students with other procedures, changes in doctors' orders as needed, etc.
11:00 – 12:00	• Give medications as ordered • Feed patient • Assess vital signs as ordered • Continue to assess client and document findings • Care for indwelling lines • Continue interventions and assess effectiveness	Assist students as needed

HOW TO STRUCTURE A TYPICAL CLINICAL DAY (cont'd)

Time	Student Activity	Instructor Reminders and Notes (The following are examples.)
Lunch	• Plan your lunch around your client's needs (you will need to cover for your fellow students)	• Schedule student and your breaks and meals around client's needs • Depending on the level of the students, i.e. if this is their first semester versus a senior nursing student, decide if they will cover for each other or go as a group
1:00 – 1:45 PM	• Continue to assess if client outcomes are being met and document • Continue client teaching and document • Complete any scheduled interventions or procedures	• Continue rounds of students' clients • Ensure students have completed their care
1:45 – 2:30 PM	• Complete final assessment and document client's progress toward outcomes • Document I & O • Record IV and other drainage • Make sure client is safe • Room is neat • Check to see if all medications have been given and documented with client responses	• Evaluate student documentation • Has the student documented the client's response to interventions and progress toward outcomes? • Do their notes include changes in the client's assessment? • Are I & O's recorded? • Are there any medications, treatments or procedures that have not been done? • Make quick rounds to ensure all patients are safe
2:30 PM	Give SBAR to the assigned nurse	Ensure all students have reported off using SBAR to the assigned nurse
2:30 – 3:00 PM	Post conference	Conduct post conference using inquiry and reflection questions (see charts in Chapter 3 for examples)
	Go home and be thankful another clinical day is over and you are one day closer to graduation! Seriously, spend some time reflecting over your experience and answer assigned reflections questions.	Go home, kick your feet up and be happy another clinical day is over! Seriously: Take time to reflect on how the day went and what you can do to improve the next clinical day with your students.

Handout 2

MEDICATION PROTOCOL: A FAIL SAFE APPROACH

1. Prior to beginning medication administration:
   a. Verify orders
   b. Gather needed client assessments (i.e., B/P, pulse, or other required assessment data)
   c. Check needed lab results (i.e., potassium level if client has lasix ordered, blood sugar or glucometer readings for insulin, drug levels)
   d. Check to see if any clients are NPO, or are going for procedures, dialysis, etc.

2. Pull the Medication Record for your client (the MAR). Do only one client at a time.
3. Obtain the medications you need (your clinical faculty may have to do this for you based on the medication system in your facility, i.e., scanners).
4. Lay your MAR on the counter and/or use the computer screen to check your medications, vials, IV piggy backs, IV fluids beside the name on the sheet.

5. Know what each of your medications is: Do you have all the information you need prior to giving the medication? If not, obtain and review this information and have it ready.
   a. Action
   b. Key side effects
   c. Nursing implications
   d. Why the client is getting the medication?
   e. Food/drug or drug/drug interactions
   f. Known allergies
   g. What do you need to teach your patient about the medication?

6. Check the medications against the MAR in order as they are listed to ensure: (leave medications in their wrappers and do not draw medications from the vials without your faculty).
   a. Do you have the right medication?
   b. Is the medication scheduled at this time?
   c. Is it the right dose?
   d. Is there any information you need prior to giving the medication, i.e., B/P readings, digoxin levels you do not have?
   e. Has the medication already been given?
   f. Based on what you know about the medication, does it make sense (rationale) that this client would be getting this medication?
   g. Is there any information that needs to be recorded on the MAR prior to giving the medication, i.e., blood pressure?

7. Let your instructor know you are ready to check off your medications.
8. Go through information listed in Step number 5 with your faculty. At this time, adjust any dosages, i.e., cut the pill, pull up the correct dose for injections.
9. Once you have completed the check-off with your faculty, take your MAR and the medications still in their wrappers (or the scanner) to the client's bedside.
10. Perform seven rights for medications, check your meds as you open them with the MAR.
11. Sign off the medications on the MAR as the client takes them and perform necessary client teaching.
12. Return the MAR to the appropriate place or scanner and note when your next medications are due. Document client teaching.
13. Evaluate client's response to medications.
14. Document client's response and progress toward outcome.

STUDENT REPORT SHEET

0700

Client Initials

Room

Safety Huddle
AM Report
System Review
Check line patency**
List treatments needed
SBAR

*Always review and note trends!

LABS :

I&Os:

VS: T° _____ BP _____ HR _____ RR _____

Sat %

Man: BP _____ HR _____ RR _____

VS: 24 hour trends:

0800

Check BS _____

24 hour BS trends _____

Give Insulin

Breakfast

Hourly Rounding

Chart: Client activity

Client Education

Med Administration

Rhythm _____ Rate _____

0900

Med Administration

Rhythm _____ Rate _____

Begin Treatments

Clinical Paperwork

Hourly Rounding

Chart: Client activity

Treatments

Ambulate

Rhythm _____ Rate _____

Clinical Paperwork

1100

Eat Lunch

Treatments

Ambulate

Rhythm _____ Rate _____

Clinical Paperwork

1200

Check BS _____

Give Insulin

Lunch

Hourly Rounding

Chart: Client activity

Rhythm _____ Rate _____

VS: T° _____ BP _____ HR _____ RR _____

Sat _____

Man: BP _____ HR _____ RR _____

*Indicate Normal/Abnormal and Report

1300

Wrap Up:

Treatments

Clinical Paperwork

Chart: I & O

*Clear Pumps

Rhythm _____ Rate _____

Give 1400 meds if assigned

Review Charting

Report off: SBAR

Post-conference Points

Created by Dr. Jada C. Quinn

Handout 4

TYPICAL DAY EVENTS
(May vary per clinical and patient needs)

When you arrive, before 6:45 AM

+ Get report from your nurse
+ Check for new orders, new meds, time of first med, check if NPO for test, which meds are they getting, AM blood sugars

7:00 – 7:20 AM Preconference

+ Take B/P and pulse
+ Give 7:30 meds, insulin (check to see if it has been given)
+ See your pt, assess quickly, check IVs, make sure they are patent and running at the right rate with the right fluid, check for any other lines, tubes that they are patent and what is draining

By 9:30 AM

+ Give meds and complete assessment or vise versa as appropriate
+ Give assessment to your nurse to enter in the computer
+ AM care (you may do part of your assessment then)

10 AM

+ Chart opening nursing note with AM assessment by_____(Time)

10:30 AM

+ Treatments or procedures ordered (This may come earlier if scheduled for tests.)
+ Do patient teaching as needed. Continue to check for new Dr.'s orders
+ Check for lab results, particularly PTT if on heparin. 11:00–12:00 check for noon BS if ordered, eat lunch, feed pt if needed

11 AM

+ Vital signs (give results to techs) Continue to assess patient's response and progress toward outcomes.

Lunch for 30 min between the hours of 11:00 and 12:00 based on your patient's needs and schedules

Give 11 and 12 o'clock meds if ordered, Flush INTs

+ Continue to reinforce patient teaching and interventions to help your patients achieve the outcomes and continuously reassess your patient

1:00 PM

+ Wrap-up, do final assessment, make sure patient is okay and room is neat
+ Do I & O (give results to techs to chart and chart results in your nurse's notes). Check to see if all meds have been given and charted.

1:30 PM

+ Chart final notes: include evaluation of your patient's progress or lack of progress toward the outcomes. How is he doing? Is he getting better? Include I & O and record again information on IVs, drains, etc.

By 2:00 PM

+ Report off to your nurse and your clinical instructor using SBAR

2:00 PM Post-conference

SHIFT REPORT USING SBAR FORMAT

The Situation and Background will only need to be entered the first time you report on this client.

Situation: Patient Name, Age, Sex

                          Room Number

                          Physician(s)

Background: Admission Diagnosis (date of surgery)

                          Past medical history that is significant (hypertension, CHF, etc)

                          Allergies

This information should be included in each report if applicable.

Assessment: Code Status (any advance directives, DNR orders, POAHC)

                          Procedures done in previous 24 hours including results/outcomes
                          (include where we stand with post procedure vitals/assessment)

                          Abnormal assessment findings

                          Abnormal vital signs

                          IV fluids/drips/site; when is site to be changed

                          Current pain score—what has been done to manage pain

                          Safety Needs—fall risk, skin risk, etc.

Recommendations: Needed changes in the plan of care (diet, activity, medication,
                          consultations)?

                          What are you concerned about?

                          Discharge planning

                          Pending labs/x-rays, etc

                          Calls out to Dr. _____about_____

                          What the next shift needs to do or be aware of—i.e., labs to be drawn in AM

NOTES

CHAPTER 3

Improving Critical Thinking and Clinical Judgment

IN THIS CHAPTER YOU WILL LEARN HOW TO:

➡ Develop inquiry questions

➡ Develop reflection questions

➡ Apply inquiry and reflection questions

➡ Use thinking strategies to develop clinical judgment

Now that you have a structure for organizing your clinical day, a protocol for medication administration, and a tool to help students organize their care, it is time to help students improve their critical thinking and clinical judgment skills. When we have worked with clinical facilities, they want their new graduate nurses to have critical thinking skills. Observation of student performance is a part of the clinical instructor role. However, observation does not give you information on what the student is thinking. Likewise, questions asked randomly without purpose lead to inconsistent outcomes. When clinical instructors use observation with questions asked in a deliberate and systematic way, it strengthens the student's critical thinking skills. We have developed two methods of questioning to help students acquire critical thinking skills and improve their ability to make clinical judgments.

DEVELOP INQUIRY QUESTIONS

Inquiry questions require the students to reveal what they know. There is a hierarchy of inquiry questions from knowledge to synthesis. It is essential for clinical instructors to ask questions that take the student beyond memorization of facts to application, analysis, and synthesis. Asking inquiry questions helps clinical instructors determine if the student knows how to give safe and effective care. This also helps students learn the kind of questions they need to ask themselves when the clinical instructor is not present. Begin the inquiry process with knowledge level questions:

✦ Does the student know the basic facts?

✦ If they know facts, have the student apply the facts to the total client's care.

✦ If they can apply the facts to the care, assist the student to make choices among options.

✦ If they are successful, ask questions that require the student to consider knowledge, past experience and the client's situation simultaneously needed to make clinical judgments.

The table below gives examples of each of these types of questions.

Types of Inquiry Questions

DEFINITIONS	EXAMPLES OF INQUIRY QUESTIONS
Knowledge: Memorized information /facts	What is the normal range for blood pressure?
Application: Connecting knowledge to a clinical situation	Which is the most important vital sign to monitor in your client who has hypertension?
Analysis: Understanding pros & cons, strengths and weaknesses or options in decision-making	In your client with a blood pressure of 95/60, should you administer the anti-hypertensive medication as ordered?
Synthesis: Pulling together multiple sources of experiences, data and information to make judgments about needed client care. This process may require several inquiry questions to guide the student.	What has the blood pressure been for the past two days? Is this the same or has there been a change? What could be contributing to this change in their B/P? Are there any guidelines in the doctor's orders regarding their B/P? What nursing actions will you take?

At the end of the chapter, **The Quick Approach: Inquiry Questions Organized Around the Nursing Process** will provide you with multiple examples of questions that you can apply in different client care situations.

DEVELOP REFLECTION QUESTIONS

Reflection questions require students to think about their own thinking. Reflection challenges students to self-monitor, plan, and revise their own thinking so they can quickly self-correct. Reflection results in safe and effective decisions about the needed client care and the prevention of complications. Reflective thinking is an essential component of clinical judgment. Clinical instructors need to role model reflective practice and the habit of self-questioning. The way you do that is to use reflection questions. Included at the end of the chapter in handout 2 is an **Example of Reflection Questions** that clinical instructors can use to reflect on their clinical experience for the day. They can be handed in at post conference or the following day. This example includes points that are a part of the **Rubric for the Outcome Web** (Chapter 4, handout 2). Reflection questions can be changed weekly and adapted to meet the needs of the clinical day. The mark of a true professional is to reflect constantly about their clinical practice

APPLY INQUIRY AND REFLECTION QUESTIONS

At the end of the chapter, handout 3, is a **Urinary Catheterization Algorithm** that displays how clinical instructors use inquiry and reflection questions before, during, and after a urinary catherization. The questions included in the algorithm help the students to see beyond the task to the clinical judgment needed even with procedures. Novice students without these questions will only approach any procedure as a task to be accomplished. Please note though, it will be important not to ask these questions during the procedure but before and after. These same types of questions apply to any procedure.

USE THINKING STRATEGIES TO DEVELOP CLINICAL JUDGMENT

Clinical judgment is not inherent in a novice thinker. In order to achieve this level of development in students' thinking, the clinical instructor needs to teach them how and once again, role modeling is the best way. You can use inquiry and reflection questions to help students adopt a structured way of thinking about a client situation. This process will help students build clinical judgment skills. The chart **Thinking Strategies to Improve Students Clinical Judgment**, at the end of the chapter, lists thinking strategies, their definitions, and use of them in clinical. The chart combines thinking strategies with inquiry and reflection questions.

NOTES

THE QUICK APPROACH: INQUIRY QUESTIONS FOR CLINICAL KNOWLEDGE ORGANIZED AROUND THE NURSING PROCESS

Assessment

1. Which vital sign assessments would be the highest priority for a client with a specific clinical diagnosis (i.e., temperature, pulse, respiratory rate, and blood pressure) and why?

2. Which of the above vital signs should be reported to a team member or provider of care and why?

3. Which assessments would be a priority for your client (i.e., BP, bradycardia, bleeding, etc.) and why?

4. What is the highest priority nursing action before initiating an order? (Check/verify accuracy of order)

5. Which assessment finding is a priority for monitoring your client's hydration status (i.e., I & O, edema, signs and symptoms of dehydration)?

6. Which of your clients should be assessed/triaged initially and why?

7. Which of the psychosocial, spiritual, cultural and occupational assessment findings may affect the client's care (i.e., cultural—dietary, occupational—stress, etc.) and why?

Analysis/Diagnosis

1. Prior to administering the medication, which data would be most pertinent to review (i.e., vital signs, lab results, allergies, etc.)?

2. When adjusting or titrating dosage of medications, what physiological parameters did you use (i.e., giving insulin according to blood sugar levels, titrating medication to maintain a specified blood pressure, etc.)?

3. Which systems-specific assessment or reassessments would be the priority for your client and why (i.e., GI, respiratory, cardiac, etc.)?

4. How will you prioritize your care based on the information you received in shift report and why?

5. Which level of nursing personnel would be most appropriate to assign to your client if you were making out assignments (i.e., LPN, VN, assistive personnel, other RNs, etc.)?

6. Which of the clients would be most appropriate to transfer to the (medical surgical unit, orthopedic, psychiatric, etc.) unit?

Outcomes

1. What clinical outcomes best determine the effect of the pain medication?

2. What assessment findings indicate an improvement in the client's hydration status?

3. What clinical findings are expected when the dopamine dosage is titrated appropriately?

4. What clinical findings are expected when the insulin is titrated according to the blood sugar levels?

5. Which assessment findings indicate a positive outcome from the albuterol (Ventolin) treatment?

6. Which assessment findings indicate positive outcomes from (specific medications)?

7. After a specific diagnostic test (i.e., cardiac catheterization, liver biopsy, stress test, etc.), and what clinical outcomes indicate a complication?

THE QUICK APPROACH: INQUIRY QUESTIONS FOR CLINICAL KNOWLEDGE ORGANIZED AROUND THE NURSING PROCESS (cont'd)

Plan

1. Which plan would be most effective for maintaining client confidentiality/privacy?

2. What steps are most important when administering medications by the oral route or gastric tube (i.e., PO, sublingual, nasogastric tube, G tube, etc.)?

3. What plan is most appropriate for preparing medication for administration (i.e., crush medications as needed and appropriate, place in appropriate administrative device, assemble equipment, etc.)?

4. What should be included in the plan to avoid when administering medications (i.e., food, fluids, and other drugs) to minimize medication interactions?

5. What nursing care is important to include in the plan for a client receiving oxygen therapy?

6. What plan is most appropriate when using equipment in performing client care procedures and treatment?

7. What is the priority plan for maintaining your client's skin integrity (i.e., skin care, turn client, etc.)?

8. Which plan would be most appropriate to protect your client from injury (i.e., falls, electrical hazards, malfunctioning equipment, rugs, clutter, etc.)?

9. Which assessment findings would result in the nurse developing a plan to collaborate with other disciplines while providing care to the client (i.e., physician, RT, PT, radiology, dietary, lab, etc.)?

10. What is the plan for assisting the client in the performance of activities of daily living (i.e., ambulation, reposition, hygiene, transfer to chair, eating, toileting, etc.)?

11. What plan is most important to develop after evaluating the risk assessment profile for your client (i.e., sensory impairment, potential for falls, level of mobility, etc.) and why?

12. How does your plan of care address the special needs of the elderly client?

Implement

1. What nursing intervention would have the highest priority for promoting infection control for your client (i.e., hand washing, appropriate room assignment, isolation, aseptic/sterile technique, universal precautions)?

2. Which nursing actions will be most appropriate with medication administration (Implement the Rights of medication administration)?

3. During an IV infusion, what is most important to monitor and maintain (i.e., infusion site, equipment, flushing infusion devices, checking, rates, fluid, and sites, etc.)?

4. What is the priority intervention for your client who is receiving medication by the intravenous route (i.e., IVP, IVPB, PCA pump, continuous infusion fluids, parenteral nutrition) or by SC, IM, intradermal or topical or in the form of eye, ear or nose drops, sprays, ointments or by inhalation (including nebulizer or metered dose inhaler)?

5. Which calculations did you use for medication administration?

6. Which health care provider orders have you received and implemented today and/or transcribed?

7. What regulations did you comply with when working with controlled substances (i.e., counting narcotics, wasting narcotics, etc.)?

8. What information did you share with the client/family regarding the medication regimen, treatments, and/or procedures?

9. Which nursing actions are most important when performing a head-to-toe assessment?

10. How did you perform the health history and how was the information utilized?

THE QUICK APPROACH: INQUIRY QUESTIONS FOR CLINICAL KNOWLEDGE ORGANIZED AROUND THE NURSING PROCESS (cont'd)

11. When communicating with your client, what is your best response?

12. What therapeutic communication techniques were used to support your client or family and/or increase client understanding of his/her behavior?

13. What interventions would be effective in assisting client with emotional and spiritual needs?

14. When performing a diagnostic test (i.e., O_2 saturation, glucose monitoring, testing for occult blood, gastric pH, urine specific gravity, etc.) what are the most important interventions?

15. Which interventions would be the highest priority to manage/prevent possible complications of your client's condition and/or procedure (i.e., circulatory complications, seizures, aspiration, potential neurological complications, etc.) or a client on a ventilator?

16. How did you act as a client advocate during the clinical experience?

17. What intervention was used to provide client and family with information about condition/illness, expected progression, and/or possible outcomes?

18. What procedures did you implement in order to admit, transfer or discharge the client?

19. What steps did you take in discontinuing or removing: IV, NG, urethral catheter, or other lines or tubes?

20. What is the appropriate nursing care for devices and equipment used for drainage (i.e., surgical wound drains, chest tube suction, or drainage devices, urethral catheter care, etc.)?

21. Which nursing intervention would be a priority for providing therapy for comfort and treatment of inflammation, swelling (i.e., apply heat and cold treatments, elevate limb, etc.)?

22. What are the appropriate steps in performing or assisting with a dressing change (i.e., wound, central line dressing, etc.)?

Evaluation

1. Which documentation is most appropriate for a procedure, treatment, or medication and what is the client's response?

2. Is the medication order appropriate for your client (i.e., appropriate for the client's condition, given by appropriate route, in appropriate dosage, etc.)?

3. What documentation in the chart indicates an understanding of the appropriate education necessary for client and family regarding pain management?

4. Which documentation evaluates teaching performed and the level of understanding of client, family or staff?

5. Which documentation indicates the client and family have been educated about his/her rights and responsibilities?

6. Which documentation indicates that the client has given informed consent for treatment?

7. What information in report indicates an understanding of priority information to include for the client(s)?

8. After a specific diagnostic test (i.e., lab, radiology, EKG, etc.), what results would be the most concern for your client?

9. After initiating the plan of care, how did you evaluate the client care (i.e., multidisciplinary care plan, care map, critical pathway, etc.)?

10. Which clinical findings indicate a need to evaluate the client's weight?

EXAMPLE OF REFLECTION QUESTIONS

Student Name _____ Clinical Instructor _____

Sec # _____   Date_____   Sat/UnSat or Grade_____

Due to Clinical Instructor: _____

12 points possible and will be added to Outcome Web Rubric Grading Sheet

1. Explain your rationale for choosing your priority nursing outcomes. (3 points)

2. Describe the relationships and/or rationales for the care, medications and/or treatments ordered and provided for your client today based on the reason for their admission to the hospital. (6 points)

3. What went well today for you in clinical and why? (1 point)

4. What would you do differently if you could and why? (1 point)

5. Today I learned . . . (1 point)

URINARY CATHETERIZATION ALGORITHM

Expected Outcome: Urinary flow established through the catheter while maintaining asepsis and patient comfort.

Inquiry and Reflection Questions about Insertion of a Foley Catheter

Why does this client need a foley? (Application)
> Possible answers: Fluid management, incontinence, post-op renal or urinary rocedures

What are potential complications for this client from having a foley? (Application)
> Possible answers: Urinary tract infections, skin irritations

What is important to monitor in this client with a foley? (Application)
> Possible answers: I & O, signs of infection, color, odor, amount of urine

What are the infection control issues for this client with a foley? (Application)
> Possible answers: Sterile procedure, potential UTI from the catheter, obtaining specimens

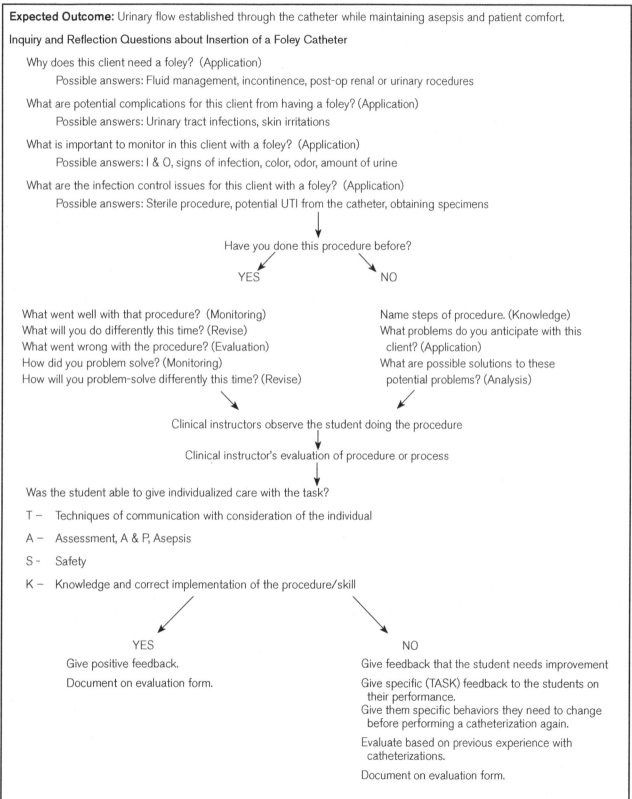

Have you done this procedure before?

YES

NO

What went well with that procedure? (Monitoring)
What will you do differently this time? (Revise)
What went wrong with the procedure? (Evaluation)
How did you problem solve? (Monitoring)
How will you problem-solve differently this time? (Revise)

Name steps of procedure. (Knowledge)
What problems do you anticipate with this client? (Application)
What are possible solutions to these potential problems? (Analysis)

Clinical instructors observe the student doing the procedure

Clinical instructor's evaluation of procedure or process

Was the student able to give individualized care with the task?

T –   Techniques of communication with consideration of the individual

A –   Assessment, A & P, Asepsis

S -   Safety

K –   Knowledge and correct implementation of the procedure/skill

YES
Give positive feedback.
Document on evaluation form.

NO
Give feedback that the student needs improvement
Give specific (TASK) feedback to the students on their performance.
Give them specific behaviors they need to change before performing a catheterization again.
Evaluate based on previous experience with catheterizations.
Document on evaluation form.

NOTES

THINKING STRATEGIES TO IMPROVE STUDENTS CLINICAL JUDGMENT

Thinking Strategies	Definitions	Faculty Strategies	Inquiry Questions Examples	Reflection Questions Examples
Knowledge Work	• Active use of reading, memorizing, drilling, writing, reviewing, and practicing to learn clinical vocabulary and facts.	• Set the structure and expectations required for preparation prior to clinical • Give clear feedback on what knowledge they need to know, i.e., drug-action of medication	• Why does a client with heart failure have edema?	• What knowledge did I need about heart failure that I did not know? • What do I need to know before I care for a heart failure client again?
Prototype Identification	• Using a model case as a reference point for comparative analysis.	• Compare students' clients to prototype in the textbooks or learned in the class room.	• How would a prototype case of congestive heart failure present?	• Were you able to recognize how your client was different from the prototype? • What changes will you make in the care you give next time?
Hypothesizing	• Generating potential options • Recognizing multiple approaches to an outcome or problem	• Have students hypothesize priority nursing diagnosis(es)/ problems, assessment data and priority interventions based on their client's medical diagnosis(es) prior to the beginning of clinical using concept mapping or care plans.	• What focused assessment data do you need to confirm or change your diagnosis(es) / problems? • Which of your proposed interventions are applicable? • Do you need to add or change other interventions?	• Was I able to identify the appropriate nursing diagnosis(es)/ problems and interventions for my client? • If yes, I confirmed my diagnosis(es)/ problems and interventions by_____. • If not, I needed to change, delete or add the following diagnoses/problems and interventions because _____.
Self-Talk	• Expressing one's thoughts to one's self	• Use self-talk (talk aloud to the students as you think about a situation/ problem) with the students.	• Talk aloud to me about how you will auscultate your client's lung sounds.	• Was I able to auscultate the lung sounds correctly; and if so, what do the sounds mean related to my care of the client?
Schema Search	• Accessing general/ specific patterns of past experiences that might apply to the current case.	• Uses talk aloud method to solicit past clinical experiences.	• How does this congestive heart failure client compare to the heart failure client you took care of last week?	• Based on your experiences with congestive heart failure clients, what patterns of care do you see?

THINKING STRATEGIES TO IMPROVE STUDENTS CLINICAL JUDGMENT (cont'd)

Thinking Strategies	Definitions	Faculty Strategies	Inquiry Questions Examples	Reflection Questions Examples
If Then Thinking	• Linking ideas and consequences together in a logical sequence	• Ask students questions about potential clinical decisions they could make and what would be the consequences of those decisions.	• If you give the medicine now, what will happen? If you hold the medication, what will happen?	• Did I make the right decision about giving/holding the medication? If not, what would I do differently next time?
Compare & Contrast	• Comparing the strengths and weaknesses of competing alternatives	• Have students identify all the priority interventions with their strengths and weaknesses.	• What would be the most effective intervention(s) to help improve this client's breathing?	• Did I choose the most effective/efficient intervention to improve my client's breathing? • If yes, I knew it was the most effective outcome because … If no, I would do what differently next time?
Trending	• Comparing the client's clinical presentation from one observation to the next observation	• Have students compare, contrast and trend their assessments of their clients they made in the beginning of the clinical with the assessments they make throughout the clinical day.	• What were the trends you identified in the assessments you made of your client? • Are there any changes in your assessment? • What actions do you need to take based on your assessment?	• Was I able to identify the trends and changes accurately? • Were your actions appropriate? • If yes, I knew because…. • If no, I would do what differently?

Nursing Concept Map

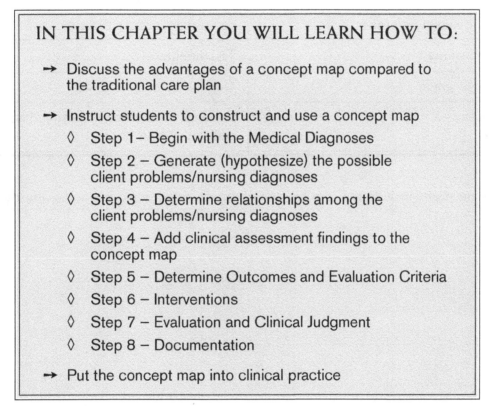

The concept map provides an excellent tool for clinical faculty to help students develop clinical reasoning skills. It is a strategy to externalize thinking, layer levels of clinical reasoning, and promote understanding of interrelationships. It is very typical for novices to focus on one particular assessment, nursing diagnoses or intervention without an understanding of the complexity and interrelationships of the care needed for the client. The concept map helps students see the full scope of the client situation and assists you to see what the student is thinking about their plan of care. The chart below compares the advantages of using the concept map compared to the traditional five-column care plan in helping the students develop clinical reasoning.

ADVANTAGES OF THE CONCEPT MAP
COMPARED TO THE TRADITIONAL CARE PLAN

Concept Map	Traditional Five-Column Care Plan
Visual picture of the interrelationships among the nursing diagnoses /problems	Nursing problems/nursing diagnoses seen in isolation
Systems approach	Linear approach
Outcome thinking	Problem thinking
Focuses on nursing priorities	Focuses on medical/disease
Decision making	Task oriented
Less time to grade	Time consuming to grade
Total pages 1–2	Depends on number of nursing diagnoses and can go on and on . . .

The following pages include the step-by-step approach to constructing and using the concept map.

HOW TO INSTRUCT STUDENTS TO CONSTRUCT AND USE A CONCEPT MAP

Students begin clinical by receiving their client assignment with the medical diagnoses. The nursing process guides the steps in the development of the concept map.

STEP 1: Place the medical diagnoses/client situation in the middle of the paper with any pertinent client history that would impact the current admission.

Med DX: CHF
Hx: Chronic
Renal Disease

STEP 2: Generate (hypothesize) the possible client problems/nursing diagnoses that might be associated with the medical diagnoses.

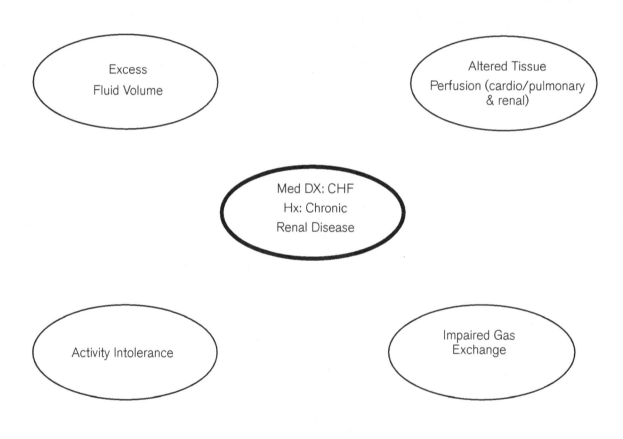

STEP 3: Determine the relationships among the client problems/nursing diagnoses. Here is what you would say to your student: *"Is there any logical reason why these two problems might be related to each other?"*

a. *"Is there any logical reason why excess fluid volume would be related to activity intolerance?"*

b. If the answer is yes, draw a line to connect them.

c. In this example, excess fluid volume leads to activity intolerance, so draw the line between excess fluid volume and activity intolerance.

d. Working systematically around the circle, you will ask yourself, *"Is excess fluid volume related to the other client's problems/nursing diagnoses included on the map?"*

e. Now ask, *"Is there any logical reason why excess fluid volume is related to impaired gas exchange?"*

f. If the answer is yes, draw a line between the excess fluid volume and impaired gas exchange.

g. In this case, excess fluid volume leads to impaired gas exchange.

h. Finally ask, *"Is there any logical reason why excess fluid volume is related to altered tissue perfusion?"*

i. If the answer is yes, draw the line between excess fluid volume and altered tissue perfusion.

j. In this example, excess fluid volume leads to altered tissue perfusion.

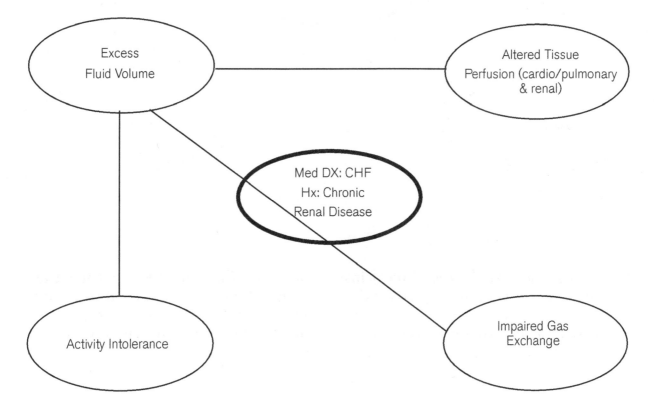

The first layer of the map is complete. We now begin with the next layer of the map.

Repeat the process for all of the nursing diagnoses listed asking the same questions about the relationships between one diagnosis and another. If the answer is yes, draw a line between the two diagnoses.

As you can see, all of these client problems/nursing diagnoses are highly interrelated. So interventions aimed at one client problem/nursing diagnoses may help with the other client problems/nursing diagnoses. The goal is to select priority interventions based on clinical assessment findings that will have the greatest impact on the client's problem.

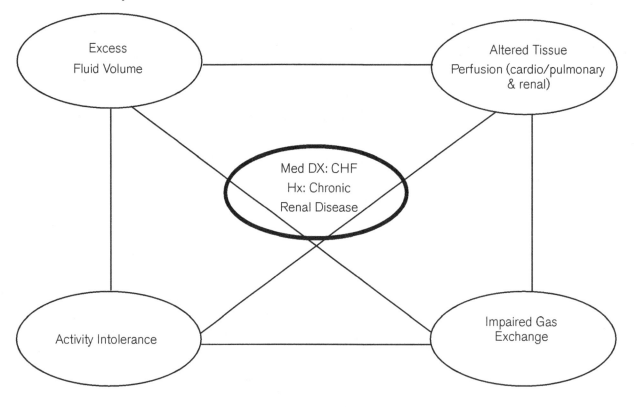

☞ *Teaching point*: As the clinical instructor, guide the students about what are priority client problems or needs and what are not. Students often want to include anxiety, risk for infection on every client's concept map. Yes, it is important for the students to assess for anxiety and take steps to prevent infection, but add these to the concept map only if clinical assessment findings support it.

STEP 4:
Add clinical assessment findings to the concept map. The following chart illustrates how assessment data are added to the concept map with the nursing diagnosis of excess fluid volume.

Defining S/SX for Excess Fluid Volume	**Actual** Clinical Assessment Findings
Weight gain >2 lbs. in 24 hours	Weight 120 lbs. yesterday, today 124 lbs.
SOB	SOB
Rales/rhonchi	Yes, R LLobe
Edema	No Edema

Each client's nursing diagnoses chosen by the students have a set of defining signs and symptoms that indicate the client nursing diagnoses. The students then complete their assessment of the client and compare their actual assessment clinical findings to the defining signs and symptoms. This comparison will tell the students if the client has the nursing diagnosis/problem or not. Students normally associate signs and symptoms with something that is wrong. The goal for the students is to focus as much attention to positive indicators as well as negative indicators. For example, if the student assesses for the defining signs and symptoms of excess fluid volume and there is no edema, it is a very important positive assessment clinical

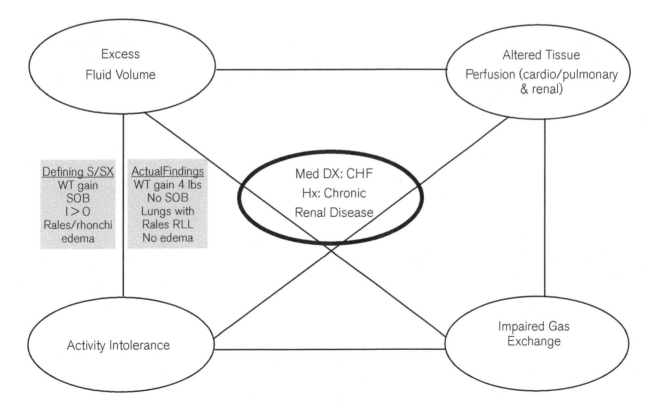

finding. It does not mean, however, you stop assessing for edema on this CHF client. The monitoring, comparing, contrasting, and trending of the clinical assessment findings leads to early identification and/or prevention of potential complications. You are teaching an expected and essential competency required of a new graduate nurse that directly impacts the safety of the client.

✏️ *Teaching Point:* After reviewing the prior data with the students, you want to evaluate if they have identified the priority clinical assessment findings for the nursing diagnosis of Excess Fluid Volume. If they, for example, left out daily weight as a priority clinical assessment finding, review with them why monitoring daily weights is the best method of determining fluid status in a client.

Assuming in this case they have included the priority clinical assessment findings, ask the following inquiry questions:

1. *"What clinical findings indicate that your client may have excess fluid volume?"*

2. *"I notice you stated the client gained 4 lbs."* Is this a weight gain over the past week or in the past 24 hours?

Let's assume for teaching purposes, the student says they do not know. Your next question would be:

3. *"Why would this be important to know if your client gained or lost weight in the past 24 hours?"*

Using these inquiry questions, you are guiding your student to see that a 4 lb. weight gain in 24 hours is a significant clinical finding and helps validate excess fluid volume. This process is repeated for all of the nursing diagnoses on the concept map.

STEP 5: Determine Outcomes and Evaluation Criteria

Setting outcomes are very difficult for students because they have so little experience. They have great difficulty with outcome focused thinking. Here is an easy way to teach students how to develop outcomes. Transform the nursing diagnosis into a positive term. For example, let's take the diagnosis, "Excess fluid volume" and ask, "What is the positive of this problem?" The answer is "Fluid Volume Balance". . . voila the **OUTCOME**!

The next step is to determine if the outcome was met and if so, how do you know that? You develop evaluation criteria using the same process where you used the assessment data and transform them into desired outcomes. For example, one of the assessments for excess fluid volume is "weight gain of 4 lbs since yesterday". The desired outcome can be measured by the evaluation criterion of "weight gain < 2 lbs per day.

The following table illustrates the outcome and evaluation criteria development process for all of the client problem/nursing diagnoses used in this example.

Determine Outcomes and Evaluation Criteria Table

Client Problem/ Nursing Diagnosis	Clinical Assessment Findings	Outcome	Evaluation Criteria
Excess fluid volume	• Weight gain 4 lbs from yesterday • Lungs with rales in left lower lobe • c/o SOB	Fluid Volume Balance	• Wt gain < 2 lbs/day • Lungs clear • No SOB • No edema
Activity Intolerance	• Increase SOB • Increase pulse from 85 to 96 BPM with activity • Pulse returns to baseline 10 min after activity	Tolerates Activity	• No SOB • Pulse within client's norm • Pulse returns to baseline < 3 min after activity
Impaired Gas Exchange	• c/o of SOB • c/o of anxiety • Respirations 23/minute • O_2 Sat 91%	Adequate Gas Exchange	• No SOB • No c/o of anxiety • Respirations 16–20/min • O_2 Sat > 95%
Altered tissue perfusion	• Capillary refill > 3 sec • Pulses + 1 • Skin cool • Color pale	Adequate tissue perfusion	• Capillary refill < 3 sec • Pulses +2 • Skin warm and dry • Color pink

STEP 6: Interventions

Now that the outcomes have been established, we can move forward with the interventions that will help achieve the outcomes. It is very important to select the best interventions to achieve the outcomes using the compare and contrast thinking strategy (Chapter 3). Using the same example client in the concept, the table below illustrates this process with the four nursing diagnoses used.

Client Problem/ Nursing Diagnosis	Clinical Assessment Findings	Outcomes	Evaluation Criteria	Interventions
Excess fluid volume	• Weight gain 4 lbs from yesterday • Lungs with rales in left lower lobe • c/o SOB • No edema	Fluid Volume Balance	• Wt gain < 2 lbs /day • Lungs clear • No SOB • No edema	• Weigh daily, compare & trend • Assess I & O • *Assess Lung sounds* • *Cough and deep breathe q 4 hrs* • *Incentive spirometer every hour while awake* • *Semi-Fowler's position* • *Assess SOB* • *Assess edema*
Activity Intolerance	• Increase SOB • Increase pulse from 85 to 96 BPM with activity • Pulse returns to baseline 10 min after activity	Tolerates Activity	• No SOB • Heart rate within client's norm • Ht rate returns to baseline < 3 min after activity	• *Assess SOB* • Teach client to pace activity • Assess pulse and RR before, during and after activity
Impaired Gas Exchange	• c/o of SOB • Lungs with rales in left lower lobe • Respirations 23/min • O_2 Sat 91%	Adequate Gas Exchange	• No SOB • Lungs clear • Respirations 16-20/min • O_2 Sat > 95%	• *Assess SOB* • Assess for restlessness • Assess RR and O_2 sat • Administer O_2 as ordered • *Assess lung sounds* • *Cough and deep breathe q 4 hrs* • *Incentive spirometer every hour while awake* • *Semi-Fowler's position*

Developing Outcomes and Evaluation Criteria With Interventions (cont'd)

Client Problem/ Nursing Diagnosis	Clinical Assessment Findings	Outcomes	Evaluation Criteria	Interventions
Altered tissue perfusion	• Capillary refill > 3 sec • Pulses + 1 • Skin cool • Color pale	Adequate tissue perfusion	• Capillary refill < 3 sec • Pulses +2 • Skin warm and dry • Color pink	• Assess cap-refill q 4 hrs • Assess pulses, color and skin temp q 4 hrs • Position with legs uncrossed • *Legs level with heart* • *Semi-Fowler's position*

Developing Outcomes and Evaluation Criteria With Interventions

The next phase in this process is to determine the priority interventions for the client. The nursing interventions *italicized* in the chart above are priority because they help achieve more than one client outcome. The other interventions are distinct to that particular nursing diagnosis and outcome. When a student sees all of the interventions on a concept map, the student is able to determine which interventions will be most effective for the most outcomes. This exercise helps the student to do system thinking and to see the whole client picture versus looking at each client problem/nursing diagnoses and outcome separately.

Teaching Point: Clinical instructors will want to use inquiry and reflection questions to help the students understand why a particular intervention would help achieve the outcome. For example, the assessment finding of rales and rhonchi in the left lower lobe indicates that the student needs to assess the lung sounds.

1. *"What intervention would help clear fluid from the lungs?"* You hope this question will lead the students to the intervention of deep breathing and coughing and incentive spirometer.

2. *"What position would best help the client to breathe easier?"* This question would guide the student to the intervention of positioning in Semi-Fowler's.

As the student progresses during the semester, increase the complexity of the inquiry questions. For example, *"What medications are the clients taking that will assist in achieving the outcomes?"*

STEP 7: Evaluation and Clinical Judgment

The next step is to determine if outcomes have been achieved. This is not a yes or no answer, but a process of comparing the evaluation criteria to the client's current clinical findings. There are three clinical judgments that are possible.

+ Outcome met

+ Outcome partially met

+ Outcome not met

Now that a decision about outcome achievement must be made, the clinical instructor needs to help the students decide what they are going to do next. What are their nursing responsibilities? This is clinical judgment. Clinical judgment uses a series of reflective questions to help make a clinical judgment about future client care as indicated in the questions below.

OUTCOME NOT MET

1. Did the client's situation change (i.e., the client had a respiratory arrest)?
   a. If yes, revise plan of care to correspond to the new client condition.
   b. If no, go on to the next question.
2. Were the interventions ineffective?
   a. If yes, revise the interventions.
   b. If no, go on to the next question.
3. Did I evaluate too soon or is more time needed for the interventions to be effective?
   a. If yes, continue the current care and continue to evaluate.
   b. If no, go to next question.
4. Were the conclusions drawn from the clinical assessment findings accurate?
   a. If yes, continue the current plan of care and continue to evaluate.
   b. If no, re-analyze the clinical assessment findings to determine correct client nursing diagnosis and outcome, and revise the plan of care.

OUTCOME PARTIALLY ACHIEVED

If the outcome was partially achieved, then the student would use similar reflection questions.

1. Is more time needed for the interventions to be effective?
    a. If yes, continue the current plan of care and continue to evaluate.
    b. If no, go to next question.
2. Are changes needed in the interventions to achieve the outcome?
    a. If yes, make the changes. Increase frequency of the interventions or add new interventions.
    b. If no, continue plan of care and ongoing evaluation.

OUTCOME ACHIEVED

1. Is the problem likely to recur without nursing interventions?
    a. If no, discontinue nursing diagnosis.
    b. If yes, go to next question.
2. Does the nursing diagnosis require the same level of intervention or vigilance?
    a. If yes, continue plan of care.
    b. If no, revise plan of care to meet current needs of client.

It is common for the student to say, "The client does not have this nursing diagnosis because they have no signs and symptoms, so I need to take it off the concept map."

It is very important that the student understand there is high risk of reoccurrence of excess fluid volume in a client with CHF and renal failure. *It would not be safe practice to quit monitoring for the clinical findings of fluid volume excess when the problem is likely to reoccur.* The prudent nurse will monitor for potential complications. Therefore, excess fluid volume would remain on the concept map. Here are two examples of inquiry questions to help guide the students in this judgment process:

1. *"Your client has CHF with renal failure; what is the risk that excess fluid volume may occur?"*
2. *"What would you want to continue to monitor to prevent complications?"*

STEP 8: Documentation

Following judgment, the student will need to document in the chart their conclusions. The concept map is a useful guide for the student while they document. It is important that documentation contain the following three pieces of information:

+ Client's response to interventions

+ Progress toward the outcomes

+ Any changes in plan of care

The concept map and the student clinical recording sheet (see Chapter 3) should provide all of the information the student needs to document accurately.

PUT THE CONCEPT MAP INTO CLINICAL PRACTICE

The development of the concept map begins when students receive their clinical assignments. If students are not able to assess the assigned client, they can still begin the concept map using the prototype case (see Chapter 3). The concept map may change after the student actually assesses their client. The table on page 41 describes how the clinical instructor helps the student put the concept map into clinical practice.

Putting the Concept Map into Clinical Practice

Student Responsibility	Clinical Instructor Responsibility	Teaching Points
1. Hypothesize potential nursing problems/nursing diagnoses around the assigned client medical diagnosis(es)and bring concept map to clinical.	• Review concept map at the beginning of clinical. • You may want the students to complete separate patho, lab and med and student clinical recording sheets while they are learning (see Chapter 3).	• Does the concept map reflect the prototype client for this diagnosis(es)? If so, go to number 3. • *Remember that the concept map will not have individualized care at this point.* • *If the concept map does not reflect appropriate hypotheses, then this is a teaching opportunity to guide the student, go to number 2*
2. If hypothesized concepts are incorrect after speaking with the clinical instructor, then edit or add to the concept map. *Hint: Use pencil initially to complete concept map. Use different color pencils for different diagnoses.* DO NOT ERASE; just put an X through the revision or change colors, so you can see the CHANGE in THINKING and LEARN from this. Do not start over!	• Guide the student to include concepts that would be part of prototype client. • After the assessment, the student can cross through what was not appropriate and add what they found. • Instruct the students not to erase and start over. Using this process, you can see the change in the student's thinking.	• *(Expectation of what student should have done will be based on level of student.)* • Important to remind students that what they did the night before was not a waste of time, but a learning process to make judgments based on their assessments and the plan of care is constantly evolving to meet the needs of the client.
3. Assess your client and revise concept map as appropriate.	• Re-evaluate the concept map as the student makes changes. • (This may be done orally during the clinical day, depending on the level of the student.)	• If student was on the right track with the concept map, but after the assessment of the client revisions were needed, it is the responsibility of the clinical instructor to help the student realize this is part of the process.

Interaction between the clinical instructor and the student is similar as the student works through each of remaining steps 3 through 7 in constructing the concept map.

The concept map is an established best practice for teaching students clinical reasoning. Using the concept map does require practice and repetition on both the part of the clinical instructor and the students. When used in each clinical through a curriculum, the concept map becomes an internalized part of the students' thinking. The students are able to transition from the written concept map to oral presentations of the concept map in their last semesters of school. Systematic thinking, once illustrated through a written concept map, becomes a critical thinking habit students will use in their clinical practice.

At the end of this chapter for your reference and use are an **Example of an Outcome Concept Map**, **Rubric for Grading the Outcome Map** (both of which can also be used with nursing diagnoses or outcomes), and a **blank Nursing Diagnosis and/or Concept Map** for you to use (pages 43-46). In addition, other clinical forms that we have found helpful and that can be adapted to your needs are included: **AIDES**, **Medication Information Form for students**, **Client History and Pathophysiology Information Sheet**, **Health History and System-Specific Assessment Tool**, and a **Lab, Diagnostic Tests, and Procedure Recording Form** (pages 48–54).

EXAMPLE OF OUTCOME CONCEPT MAP

Name _____   Clinical Faculty _____   Sec # _____   Date _____   Grade _____

Nursing Diagnosis: Ineffective breathing patterns

Outcome: Client will achieve optimal respiratory function

System-Specific Assess	Outcome Desired	Interventions
1. c/o of SOB	1. No SOB	1. HOB ↑
2. RR– 26	2. RR 16–20	2. C & DB q 4 hrs
3. Rales LL bilaterally	3. Lungs clear	3. O_2 @ 2L NC
4. O_2 Sat > 95%	4. O_2 Sat > 95%	4. O_2 Sat q 4 hrs/note changes
		5. Auscultate lungs q 4 hrs

Nursing Diagnosis: Activity Intolerance

Outcome: Client will improve and/or maintain activity tolerance

System-Specific Assess	Outcome Desired	Interventions
1. RR & P↑ with activity	1. RR & P return to norm within 3 min of activity	1. Monitor RR & P before and after activity
2. c/o of SOB with activity	2. No SOB with activity	2. Teach pursed-lip breathing with activity
3. Not pacing activity	3. Pace activity	3. Teach to prioritize and pace activity
4.	4.	4.

Medical DX CHF and Pertinent History Diabetes

Nursing Diagnosis: Excess fluid Balance

Outcome: Client will maintain fluid balance

System-Specific Assess	Outcome Desired	Interventions
1. Wt gain 5 lbs/24 hrs	1. Wt within 2 lbs of norm	1. Daily wt & compare
2. I = 1240 cc > O	2. I = O	2. Monitor I & O q 8 hrs
3. Rales LL bilaterally	3. Lungs clear/no SOB	3. O_2 @ 2L NC
4. 2+edema bilaterally in LL legs	4. ↓ to no edema	4. Legs position lower than heart ROM or walking
		5. Monitor edema q 4 hrs & compare

Nursing Diagnosis: Knowledge Deficit of Low Na Diet

Outcome: Client will know how to maintain a Low Na Diet

System-Specific Assess	Outcome Desired	Interventions
1.	1.	1.
2.	2.	2.
3.	3.	3.
4.	4.	4.

Handout 1

EXAMPLE OF OUTCOME CONCEPT MAP, PAGE 2

Name _____

1. **Outcome: Client will achieve optimal respiratory function**
   Client response to interventions:
   1. HOB ↑, Pt stated ↓SOB and was able to breath without labor
   2. O$_2$ 2 l/cannula cont, O$_2$ sat 98%
   3. Lungs Rales↓ in R lobe, remain in Llower lobe

   Clinical Judgment: Was overall outcome met   Yes _____   Partially   x _____   Not at all _____

   Why (Rationale, explain your judgment): What would you do differently?

   Continue current interventions. Saw improvement in adventitious lung sounds, but still has productive cough and rales remain in Left lower lobes. Positioning and O$_2$ decreased SOB and Increase O$_2$ Sat.

2. **Outcome: Client will maintain fluid balance**
   Client response to interventions:
   1.
   2.
   3.
   4.

   Clinical Judgment: Was overall outcome met?   Yes _____   Partially   x _____   Not at all _____

   Why (Rationale, explain your judgment): What would you do differently?

3. **Outcome: Client will improve and/or maintain activity tolerance**
   Client response to interventions:
   1.
   2.
   3.
   4.

   Clinical Judgment: Was overall outcome met?   Yes _____   Partially   x _____   Not at all _____

   Why (Rationale, explain your judgment): What would you do differently?

PRIORITY LAB/PROCEDURES	RESULTS/INTERPRETATIONS	NURSING INDICATIONS (PRE & POST)
1. Electrolytes, NA & K	Na – 138mEq/L K – 3.2mEq/L	Notify Dr. prior to giving Lasix because of low K
2. Blood Sugar, HbA1c	HbA1c – 7%	Continue insulin as ordered/monitor for effect
3. BUN/Creat	BUN 19/ Creat 1.9	Continue to monitor because of CHF, diabetes and receiving ace inhibitor

RUBRIC FOR OUTCOME CONCEPT MAP

Student Name _____ Clinical Instructor _____ Date _____ Grade _____

Directions: Complete one **Nursing Outcome Concept Map** each week. You will get a Pass/Fail. One of the written outcome concept maps will be graded and one will be presented orally to your clinical instructor on designated weeks. The average of the two will be 5% of your application grade. You will receive your assigned client and primary medical diagnosis(es) when you arrive for clinical. Get the client report, do your assessment and then do the first page of the outcome concept map. The outcome concept map is a working tool, so **make appropriate changes/additions through the day as the clinical situation dictates. Use a different color ink or pencil color to make changes in the concept map.** You are to complete the first page of your concept map by the end of the clinical and your clinical instructor will review and sign. The final review will be completed when all components of the concept map, 2 medication AIDES sheets and reflection page are turned in/emailed to your faculty. SBAR will be given according to resource on blackboard or per unit protocol.

CONCEPT MAP COMPONENTS WITH CRITERIA FOR GRADING	POINTS EARNED/ POINTS POSSIBLE PASS/FAIL	CONCEPT MAP COMPONENTS WITH CRITERIA FOR GRADING	POINTS EARNED/ POINTS POSSIBLE PASS/FAIL
1. Based on the patient's medial diagnoses, draw a nursing outcome concept map **using 3 priority outcomes,** one of which should be a teaching and discharge outcome. *2 points for each of the three outcomes that are a priority 2 x 3 = 6*	____/6 ____ P/F	6. **State if outcomes were met and make a judgment about each outcome based on your evaluation** (i.e., continue, modify, discontinue) and why. *2 points for each outcome judgment x 3 = 6*	____/6 ____ P/F
2. Identify at least **4 measurable assessments and assessment findings for each outcome.** Write them under the appropriate outcome on the concept map. *2 points for each assessment and assessment finding, 8 points per outcome x 3 outcomes = 24*	____/24 ____ P/F	7. **Interpreted correctly 3 priority lab values** related to the patient's current clinical conditions with **nursing indications.** *2 points per each correctly interpreted lab value and nursing indications x 3 = 6*	____/6 ____ P/F
3. Identify at least **3 priority nursing interventions that will help achieve each outcome.** Write them beside the assessment findings under the nursing outcome concept map. **Note: Must include at least 2 action interventions** (i.e., cough & deep breathe every 2 hours **and 2 priority assessments for monitoring** the client's response (i.e., monitor VS every 4 hours and compare to previous finding). *1 point per intervention per outcome if appropriate & meet criteria*	____/12 ____ P/F	8. **Describe 2 medications and identify nursing indications and expected client response for each of the three medications.** *3 points for each medication (1 point for indication and 2 points for expected response) 2 x 3 = 6*	____/6 ____ P/F
4. **Use lines to show the relationships** between the outcomes. Different colored pencils for each outcome to draw the lines can make the relationships clearer. *Points based on relationships being valid*	____/6 ____ P/F	9. **Critical Thinking/Reflection Questions** are answered completely and clearly with appropriate detail. **See Reflection page.** *12 available points*	____/12 ____ P/F
5. On second page of concept map clearly **evaluate the client's response to each of the interventions and progress toward meeting outcomes.** *1 point for each of the evaluation responses for the intervention. 4 points/outcome x 3 = 12*	____/12 ____ P/F 100	10. **Correctly prepare and give SBAR report to clinical instructor prior to reporting off to the assigned RN.** *10 points possible*	____/10 ____ P/F 100
Total Points Possible		**Total Points Received**	

Handout 3

NURSING DIAGNOSIS AND/OR OUTCOME CONCEPT MAP TOOL

Name _____   Clinical Instructor _____   Sec # _____   Date _____   Grade _____

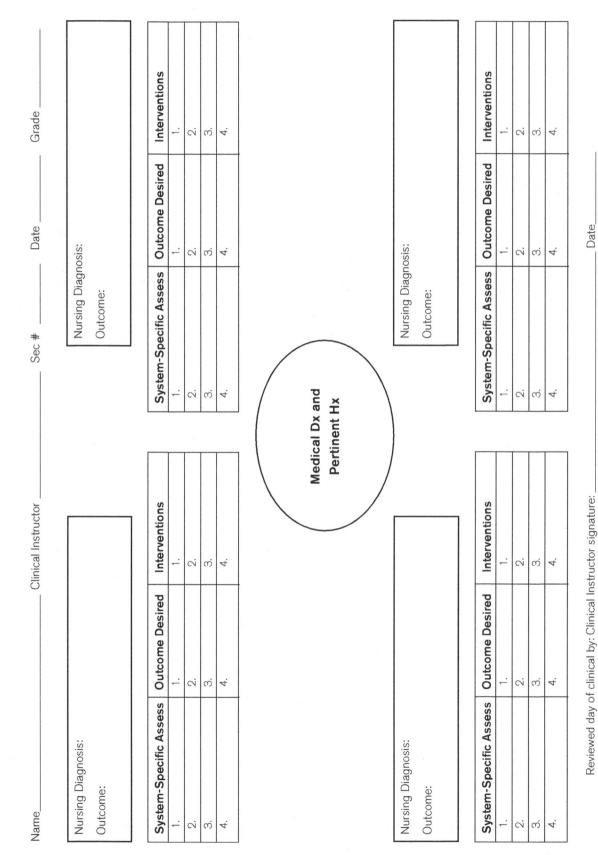

Nursing Diagnosis:
Outcome:

System-Specific Assess	Outcome Desired	Interventions
1.	1.	1.
2.	2.	2.
3.	3.	3.
4.	4.	4.

Nursing Diagnosis:
Outcome:

System-Specific Assess	Outcome Desired	Interventions
1.	1.	1.
2.	2.	2.
3.	3.	3.
4.	4.	4.

Medical Dx and Pertinent Hx

Nursing Diagnosis:
Outcome:

System-Specific Assess	Outcome Desired	Interventions
1.	1.	1.
2.	2.	2.
3.	3.	3.
4.	4.	4.

Nursing Diagnosis:
Outcome:

System-Specific Assess	Outcome Desired	Interventions
1.	1.	1.
2.	2.	2.
3.	3.	3.
4.	4.	4.

Reviewed day of clinical by: Clinical Instructor signature: _____   Date _____

NURSING DIAGNOSIS AND/OR OUTCOME CONCEPT MAP TOOL, PAGE 2

Name _____

1. Outcome:

Patient response to interventions:

1.

2.

3.

4

Clinical Judgment: Was overall outcome met?   Yes _____   Partially _____   Not at all _____

Why (Rationale, explain your judgment): What would you do differently?

2. Outcome:

Patient response to interventions:

1.

2.

3.

4.

Clinical Judgment: Was overall outcome met?   Yes _____   Partially _____   Not at all _____

Why (Rationale, explain your judgment): What would you do differently?

PRIORITY LAB/PROCEDURES   RESULTS/INTERPRETATIONS   NURSING INDICATIONS (PRE & POST)

1.

2.

3.

AIDES MEDICATION INFORMATION FORM

Directions: Please complete on _____ of your priority medications

Turn into clinical instructor _____

Have ready as information for all drugs you are administering (book, drug cards)

"AIDES" to Assist in Remembering Facts for Medication Administration

Name of Drug: Brand_____   **Generic**_____
Classification_____

A   Action of medication:

Administration of medication. Dosage ordered_____

How to administer:

Assessment:

Adverse Effects. List significant ones:

Accuracy/Appropriateness of order. Is it indicated based on client's condition, known allergies, drug-drug or drug-food interactions? If not, what action did you take?

I   Interactions (Drug-Drug, Food-Drug):

Identify priority plan prior to giving drug (i.e., vital signs, labs, allergies, etc.):

Identify priority plan after giving drug:

D   Desired outcomes of the drug:

Discharge teaching—Administration considerations for client and family:

E   Evaluate signs and symptoms of complications. Intervene if necessary and describe:

S   Safety (client identification, risk for falls, vital sign assessments):

REFERENCE:

HISTORY AND PATHOPHYSIOLOGY INFORMATION

Student Name _____ Faculty _____Sec #_____

Date _____ Pass/Fail or Grade_____

Directions: Complete and email to clinical instructor by _____.
(10 points possible on graded web noted on Rubic for Outcome web)

Client's Story (History)—What brought him/her to the hospital?

PATHOPHYSIOLOGY

Please describe the etiology (cause) and pathophysiology in your words. This is to be completed for the major diagnosis and any other active diagnoses that affect care (i.e., diabetes).

List the signs and symptoms of the disease from the textbook. Compare it to the clinical system specific assessment findings from your client (may complete the comparison after you care for your client during clinical).

Assessment findings (signs & symptoms)   Assessment findings my client manifested:
from textbook:

_____   _____

_____   _____

_____   _____

_____   _____

_____   _____

_____   _____

_____   _____

HEALTH HISTORY AND SYSTEM-SPECIFIC ASSESSMENT TOOL

Demographic Information	
Source of History	
Chief Concern/Complaint	
History of Present Illness (HPI)	
Past Medical History (PMH)	
Family History (FH)	
Social History (SH)	
Health Promotion Behaviors	
Review of Systems (ROS) System-Specific as indicated by client condition: • Integument • Head and Neck • Eyes • Ears, Nose, Mouth and Throat • Breasts • Respiratory • Cardiovascular • Gastrointestinal • Genitourinary • Musculoskeletal • Neurological • Mental Health • Endocrine • Allergic/Immunologic	
Focused History of Symptom • Location • Quality • Quantity • Timing • Setting • Alleviating or Aggravating Factors • Associated Phenomenon	

Adapted by Ellen Synovec, MN and Ellen Adkins, BSN

II PHYSICAL ASSESSMENT

General Survey
1. Appearance
2. Level of Consciousness
3. Behavior/Affect
4. Posture/dress
5. Signs of discomfort or distress
6. Assess pupils for symmetry, shape, reactivity light

Skin Assessment:
1. Color
2. Condition—Look behind ears, skin folds, between toes, soles of feet, pressure areas on shoulder, sacrum, heels
   Presence or absence or lesions, scars, wounds or piercings
3. Texture
4. Temperature
5. Skin turgor sternum
6. Nails condition, presence of clubbing
7. Capillary refill bilaterally fingers

Respiratory Assessment
1. Rate
2. Rhythm
3. Accessory muscle use
4. Chest shape and symmetry/spinal deformities/AP: LA
5. Ausculation 12 sites anterior, posterior and axillary—assess for presence or absence of adventitious sounds, cough, congestion

Cardiac assessment
1. PMI—assess location and size
2. 4 auscultation sites with diaphragm and bell
   a. Aortic—2nd RICS RSB
   b. Pulmonic—2nd LICS LSB
   c. Tricuspid—4th LICS, along left lateral sternal border
   d. Mitral or apical pulse—5th LICS MCL, apex of heart
3. Carotids—assess pulse quality, presence or absence of thrills/bruits, bilaterally
4. JVD
5. Lymph

Abdomen
1. Size
2. Shape
3. Symmetry
4. Condition—presence or absence of piercings, scars, striae, pulsations, peristalsis or bulges
5. Bowel sounds—assess all 4 quads, # sounds per minute RLQ
6. Assess for distention or tenderness with light palpation

Extremities
1. Capillary refill to UE
2. Assess UE and LE for general range of motion
3. Assess UE and LE for condition, color, temperature and presence of edema
4. Palpation of peripheral pulses—radial and dorsal pedalis
5. Assess clonus

Adapted by Ellen Synovec, MN and Ellen Adkins, BSN

Handout 7

LAB & DIAGNOSTIC TESTS AND PROCEDURES FORM

Use as Weekly Reference

Name: _____

Date: _____

Client Initials: _____

Directions: Identify all pertinent labs to the client condition, whether normal or abnormal. Describe what caused the client to have an abnormal lab or why a lab may now be normal (e.g., norm WBC–client on antibiotics). Also explain why you would or would not call the MD about this lab. These laboratory values may vary in textbooks. Look at the accepted norms for the institution where the test is interpreted to determine abnormal versus normal. This list is not all inclusive.

Lab Test	Date of Lab Test	Results	Normal	Pertinence to Client	Would You Call the MD?
Hematology					
WBC			$5.0 - 10.0\ 10^3$ ul		
RBC			$4.2 - 5.4\ 10^6$ µL		
HGB			12.0 – 16.0 g/dL		
HbA1c			6% or less		
HCT			37.0 – 47.0%		
MCV			$81 - 89\ \mu m^3$		
MCH			26 – 35 pg/cell		
MCHC			31 – 37 g/dl		
Platelets			150,000– 400,000/mm^3		
Neutrophils			37 – 75%		
Lymphocytes			19 – 48%		
Monocytes			0 – 10%		
Eosinophils			1 – 3%		
Basophils			0.0 – 1.5%		
Chemistry					
Sodium			135 – 145 mEq/L		
Potassium			3.5 – 5.1 mEq/L		
Chloride			98 – 107 mEq/L		
Glucose–serum			70 – 110 mg/dL		
Magnesium			1.3 – 2.1 mEq/L		
BUN			6 – 20 mg/dL		
Creatinine			0.7 – 1.4 mg/dL		
Calcium			8.5 –11.0 mg/dL		
Protein			6.0 – 8.0 mg/dL		
Albumin			3.5 – 5.0 mg/dL		
A/G Ratio			1.5:1.0 – 2.5 :1.0		
Total Bilirubin			0.3 –1.3 mg/dL		
Direct bilirubin			0 – 0.4 mg/dL		
Indirect Bilirubin			0.2 – .8 mg/dL		
ALT, SGPT			10 – 30 U/L		
AST, SGOT			8 – 46 U/L		

Lab Test	Date of Lab Test	Results	Normal	Pertinence to Client	Would You Call the MD?
LDH – serum			91 – 180 mg/dL		
Alk Phos			35 – 142 U/L		
Uric Acid			2 – 7 mg/dL		
Phosphorus			2.5 – 4.5 mg/dL		
Total Cholesterol			< 200 mg/dL		
LDL age > 45 (LD)			90 – 185 mg/dL		
HDL			40 – 65 mg/dL		
Triglyceride			35 – 150 mg/dL		
Urinalysis					
Color			Clear Yellow		
Appearance			Clear		
Glucose			Neg.		
Bilirubin			Neg		
Ketones			Neg		
Specific Gravity			1.015 – 1.025		
Blood			Neg		
Ph			5 – 9		
Protein			Neg		
Urobilinogen			0.5 – 4.0 mg/24hr		
Nitrates			Neg		
ABG's					
pH			7.35 – 7.45		
pCO_2			35 – 45 mm Hg		
pO_2			80 – 100 mm Hg		
HCO_3			22 – 26 mEq /L		
O_2 Sat			> 95%		
Type of O_2 client receiving					
Digoxin			0.5 – 2.0 µg/ml		
Dilantin			10 – 20 µg/ml		
Tegretol			4 – 12 µg/ml		
Theophylline			10 – 20 µg/ml		
Pt			12 – 14 SEC		
Ptt			30 – 45 SEC		
Amylase			25 – 125 U/dL		
Cardiac Enzymes					
Myoglobin			30 – 90 ng/ml		
Total CPK (CK)			Male 5 – 55 U/L Female 5 – 25 U/L		
CPK-MB			0 – 7% of total CPK		
CPK-BB			0% of total CPK		
CPK-MM			5 – 70% of total CPK		
Troponin I Value			< 0.6 ng/ml		
BNP			< 100 pg/ml		

DIAGNOSTIC TESTS/PROCEDURES

1. X-Ray, Endoscopy, Scans, Biopsy, C & S, or other special procedure reports

    Test: _____

    Date: _____

Conclusion/Interpretations: _____

    _____

    _____

Pertinence to Client: _____

2. X-Ray, Endoscopy, Scans, Biopsy, C&S, or other special procedure reports

    Test: _____

    Date: _____

Conclusion/Interpretations: _____

    _____

    _____

Pertinence to Client: _____

3. X-Ray, Endoscopy, Scans, Biopsy, C & S, or other special procedure reports

    Test: _____

    Date: _____

Conclusion/Interpretations: _____

    _____

    _____

Pertinence to Client: _____

CHAPTER 5

Interactive Strategies for Clinical Teaching

> ## IN THIS CHAPTER YOU WILL:
>
> ➡ Explore methods to create a positive clinical learning environment
>
> ➡ Examine interactive teaching strategies

While clinical can be anxiety-producing to both the clinical instructor and the students, it can also be fun. Remember the word **GAME** to help you select teaching strategies for your students.

G – Group and Team Work

A – Active Learning

M – Meaningful Partnerships

E – Eliminate Passive Learning

G - GROUP AND TEAM WORK

Today's generation of students see learning as social activity and feel it should be fun as well. Clinical provides an optimal opportunity to capitalize on team work. Working in pairs is a very effective way to help the novice clinical student gain confidence as they rely on each other's strengths and knowledge. Clinical instructors can encourage the students to use each other when they need to problem solve. Learning how to build cohesive teams in clinical is very important as peer support is a major variable in positive job satisfaction and patient safety when they enter the work force.

A – ACTIVE LEARNING

The most effective way to learn is through the active engagement with the content. This is true of both knowledge and psychomotor skills. Although today's students are skilled in accessing information instantly through the internet, they have limited ability to distinguish what is reliable versus unreliable. The clinical instructor's role is to create an environment where the students must find the information independently and make decisions about how that information would be applied in clinical. As novices learn, they just want you to tell them the answer. Clinical instructors have to set the expectation at the beginning of clinical that learning how to acquire information is a competency needed in the professional nurse. Because they are novice learners, this is going to take reinforcement and role modeling by the clinical instructor ... you have to resist just giving them the answer so they can begin to learn on their own. Clinical is the perfect place for this to occur.

M – MEANINGFUL PARTNERSHIPS

Our students today thrive in an environment where they have a meaningful partnership with their clinical instructor. They want to perceive that their instructor is a partner in their learning. They do not respond to an authoritarian approach but become engaged when you share your clinical stories. There is an extensive discussion of learning partnerships in Chapter 6.

E – ELIMINATE PASSIVE LEARNING

Clinical is an active learning environment, but as we discussed above, the clinical instructor has to help provide activities that put the student in the driver's seat for learning. Engaging students in simulation scenarios, case studies, and stories of real-life experiences can help eliminate passive learning. For example, case studies can be posted that require students to edit or add nursing interventions specific to the client-scenario using wiki software. This could be an ongoing case study in real-time, incorporating new clinical information and skills learned in clinical or in the classroom. This provides an excellent opportunity to connect the nursing concepts learned in the classroom to clinical learning and fully engage students. The interactive clinical teaching strategies listed below are other ways you can engage your students in active learning.

Interactive Clinical Teaching Strategies

Game	Description	Use
Scavenger Hunt	• Work in groups of 2 or 3 • Locate items on a unit and describe their exact location • Each group will take the others to the location	• Helpful during clinical orientation to identify location of essential equipment, supplies
Skill Day	• A planned clinical day for clinical skill review	• Can use early each semester to review new, previously learned and/or practice clinical skills
Clinical Scene Investigation—CSI	• Identify a mystery, unknown clinical fact, and/or dilemma such as "why is the patient suddenly itching?" • With your assistance, have the student(s) generate a list of possible explanations, such as drug-drug interactions, allergy, contact dermatitis, etc. • Then have the student(s) investigate the different explanations until they arrive at a conclusion, or realize they do not have enough data to solve the mystery	• Helps students seek out needed information • Also helpful for group learning • (Hint: This is a great strategy when you do not know the answer!)
Deck of Doom	• Card Game that reviews a clinical situation on a card • Give a card to the student • The student has to answer and report back to the group at post conference • An example may include the following: The client's blood sugar at 1 PM is 47; what are the priority nursing interventions for this client?	• Post conference game, or to be used for fun during the clinical day • Use to reinforce learning, such as hard-to-remember concepts, like the onset, peak times of different insulins • Use in the classroom for new information or test review
Leading Learning for the Day	• A nursing student is paired with another student to assist with clinical learning. The student leader can be assigned to a group of students	• Helpful confidence builder • Helps develop leadership, teambuilding and collaboration skills • Helpful to use when the clinical situation is very busy • Beneficial exercise during senior semesters

Interactive Clinical Teaching Strategies (cont'd)

Game	Description	Use
War Stories	• Clinical instructors or students share clinical experiences that can be positive or negative or even funny • Who can tell the best story?	• Connections between reality-based practice with theoretical learning • Stories are a vivid personal teaching method that students can connect with • Stories may involve both positive and negative clinical experiences • Ice breaker for a new clinical group • Bonding experience among clinical group and clinical instructors • A reflection exercise for the end of the semester
Who Wants to be a Millionaire?	• When asking students questions in a group about information that they are expected to know like during medication administration, give them the choice of life lines to answer the question • They can answer the question themselves • They can ask another student (call a friend) • They can ask the group (poll the audience) and choose to agree or disagree with the answer	• This is a great strategy to reduce the tension • Preserves dignity of the student • Reinforce content while still holding the students accountable for their learning • For example, can be used prior to medication administration, procedures, post conference and/or the classroom

CHAPTER 6

Collaborating With Multi-Generational Learners

IN THIS CHAPTER YOU WILL LEARN ABOUT:

→ Traditionalists and Baby Boomers as clinical instructors

→ Characteristics of Generations X and Y students

→ Teaching strategies for Generations X and Y

When you combine the characteristics of a novice learner (Chapter 1) with the characteristics of Generations X and Y, it is apparent that we cannot teach current students the way we were taught. Generational differences in characteristics, values, and learning styles are a challenge for clinical instructors when we realize our old methods of teaching may need an update. It is particularly important to know how novice learners think and learn when teaching Generations X and Y. Often, the majority of clinical instructors are Baby Boomers, with a few Traditionalists and Generation Xs, but the majority of our students are Generations X and Y (Millennial).

TRADITIONALISTS AND BABY BOOMERS AS CLINICAL INSTRUCTORS

There are challenges and opportunities for clinical instructors who are Baby Boomers. First of all, Baby Boomer clinical instructors have had to learn new technology and accept that tried and true ways do not always work. It is hard to adapt to less-is-more in communicating with Generations X and Y. Clinical instructors need to focus on what the students need to know versus what is nice to know.

CHARACTERISTICS OF GENERATIONS X AND Y STUDENTS

Generations X and Y are culturally diverse. They want balance in life; they like informality and to have fun; are highly independent and good problem solvers, but ironically require frequent feedback. They have been raised with high expectations that can lead to unrealistic perceptions of themselves and clinical instructors. The students want to know why they need to learn "this?" They prefer concrete, specific information. Generations X and Y desire personal interaction with the clinical instructor and want to be a partner in the learning process.

They are technologically literate, creative, and grew up multi-tasking…talking on the cell phone while working on the computer, and doing their homework. However, it is impossible to think about more than one thing at a time. In fact, what they do is toggle back and forth between the subjects. The danger is students then have difficulty learning anything in depth. It is a challenge for clinical instructors to turn off the toggle switch in their students and help them do outcome focused thinking.

TEACHING STRATEGIES FOR GENERATIONS X AND Y

There are important teaching strategies that clinical instructors need in developing partnerships for learning with Generations X and Y students. The word **COACH** can help clinical instructors successfully work with them.

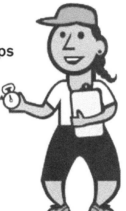

C – Collaborate and Create Partnerships

O – Off with the Toggle Switch

A – Acquire the Knowledge

C – Communication

H – Have to Give Frequent Feedback

C – COLLABORATE AND CREATE PARTNERSHIPS

As a clinical instructor you can create a positive clinical learning environment. Learning occurs best in an environment that feels safe and trusting to the student. This environment can be created by clinical instructors in numerous ways; treating students with respect, treating students equitably, speaking in a calm, controlled voice, returning clinical papers in a timely manner and giving frequent feedback in a constructive way. There are many other ways, but all of these help establish a trusting partnership between you and your students.

Generations X and Y do not view the instructor as the only one with the information or in power. They respect the clinical instructor as an expert, but they want you to partner with them in the learning process. It is still the responsibility of the clinical instructor to set expectations, adhere to standards of practice and safety, but it is not ok to be authoritarian or demeaning. You can say what you mean and mean what you say, but it is never ok to be mean. The students expect to be respected as learners and want to be included in the decisions about their learning. These decisions include being able to make choices, ask questions, express opinions and challenge, "why are we doing it this way," without fear of retribution. Rather than viewing questions as a threat to you as a clinical instructor, this is an excellent opportunity to introduce or reinforce evidence-based practice. Strong interpersonal skills are essential for successful partnerships.

O – OFF WITH THE TOGGLE SWITCH

Generations X and Y students are adept with multi-tasking, however multi-tasking is the toggling between one activity to another at a very rapid pace. Generations X and Y's ability to be on the cell phone, texting, and "Googling" information—all while they are doing their concept map—is impressive. Their ability to access large amounts of information is a great skill to have, but unfortunately this can be overwhelming. Clinical instructors need to help students prioritize what is important. With so many distracters competing for our students' attention, strategies for turning off the "toggle switch" and focusing on one topic in depth is imperative. Strategies introduced in other chapters that can help are:

+ Set expectations

+ Establish structure

+ Teach what they need to know in the moment

+ Repetition, repetition, repetition

+ Use inquiry and reflection questions

+ Model thinking strategies

These strategies will encourage critical thinking beyond the knowledge level to develop the clinical reasoning skills required of nurses today.

A – ACQUIRE THE KNOWLEDGE

Critical thinking and clinical reasoning are the desired outcomes for students in clinical. However, you cannot think about nothing, so it is essential that students acquire the base knowledge that they need. Knowledge acquisition begins in the classroom, but the true learning occurs when it is applied in clinical. The clinical instructor is charged with bringing knowledge from the classroom to clinical. This is observed through the students' ability to construct a concept map, skill in assessing, nursing interventions, medication administration, procedures, and following healthcare provider orders.

While the students are very familiar with advancing technology such as computers and smart phones, their use of this technology has been primarily for social networking. Now they need to learn how to use this technology to acquire essential knowledge needed to give safe and effective care that is based on good critical thinking and clinical decision making that achieves desired outcomes. The use of smart phones in clinical and the availability of eBooks allow the students to have instant access to needed information. Clinical instructors need to instill in the students the desire to seek current, evidence-based information. An example is to teach students how to access discipline-specific databases, such as CINAHL or MEDLINE, versus just seeking information through the Internet. Creativity, such as the strategies described in Chapter 5, can help instill the desire for students to be fully engaged in the learning process.

C –COMMUNICATION

Generations X and Y tend to communicate cryptically because of their extensive time spent on electronic communication. They have been emailing, instant messaging, and now tweeting and twittering, with family, friends, and people from different countries through the Internet; but that is very different than interpersonal communication from one person to another in the same room! This can be as simple as how to address different generations, for example, the need to address traditionalists formally with Mr. or Ms. or Sir; to being able to relate informally with Generations X and Y clients. Knowledge of interpersonal as well as therapeutic communication skills by students will make a significant difference in their ability to establish rapport with clients and the healthcare team.

Strategies to help students improve their communication skills are very important. Here are some suggestions to use during clinical:

+ Interactive role-playing and practice

+ Interpretation of non-verbal client behaviors

+ Role modeling appropriate therapeutic communication

+ Feedback about student interactions with clients

+ Simulation scenarios on effective communication

Communication is an essential skill, best learned in clinical, that impacts the therapeutic relationship the students have with their clients, and is a major factor in patient safety.

H – HAVE TO GIVE FREQUENT FEEDBACK

Generations X and Y are at home in a technological world. They grew up with interactive computer games, Nintendo, X-Box and Wii, and expect immediate feedback about how they are doing. Unlike Traditionalists and Baby Boomers, these two generations expect feedback on a frequent basis. Without frequent feedback, students have difficulty proceeding in the learning process or will incorrectly assume they are right. As a Baby Boomer clinical instructor, it is very easy for there to be a difference in perception between you and the student about their performance. The student may perceive the information as they just need to adjust, and the clinical instructor means this is not correct or acceptable, and the student needs to change behaviors immediately. Generations X and Y need explicit feedback on exactly what you as the clinical instructor want to happen. It cannot be left to interpretation. Feedback and/or counseling needs to be stated and written with clear consequences if the behavior does not change. It is very important for clinical instructors to communicate to students when they can expect to receive feedback. Mid-semester and final evaluations are not adequate to meet the needs of Generations X and Y where instant feedback is the norm. For specific strategies about giving feedback, see Chapter 7, **Assessment and Evaluation**.

NOTES

Assessment and Evaluation

IN THIS CHAPTER YOU WILL LEARN ABOUT:

➡ Establishing criteria for clinical evaluation

➡ Using feedback effectively

➡ Implementing the evaluation process and documentation

One of the most challenging aspects of being a clinical instructor is the evaluation of students. You have the responsibility of judging whether the student is able to give safe and effective care at their current level, and is able to move forward to the next semester or to graduation. This is a huge responsibility. In this chapter we will describe the process of creating an environment conducive for positive and effective evaluation of students' clinical performance.

Evaluation is the ongoing process of observing, measuring, and judging students' progress toward achievement of clinical performance outcomes. Students need to know what evaluation criteria will be used and what the consequences will be if they do not meet the criteria. Effective evaluation will:

✦ Improve skills and abilities

✦ Motivate student development

✦ Achieve student outcomes

ESTABLISHING CRITERIA FOR CLINICAL EVALUATION

The first step is to determine expectations and clinical outcomes. The course syllabus must define the expected student clinical outcomes with clear measurable evaluation criteria. There are two levels of evaluation that are ongoing in clinical evaluation. These decisions about evaluation criteria need to be made by your faculty team, outlined clearly in the syllabus or the student hand book, and students must be held accountable for this information. Holding students accountable results in prepared students and is less time consuming for the clinical instructor.

Another area requiring evaluation is student behaviors that violate patient safety standards. Your syllabus must define what constitutes unsafe care practices. These need to include but are not limited to:

✦ Failure to follow the 7 Rights of Medication Administration

✦ The number and nature of medication errors that will be allowed as part of the learning process

✦ Failure to follow infection control standards

✦ Failure to follow patient safety standards

✦ Failure to adhere to HIPPA laws

✦ Failure to report important clinical information in a timely manner to the clinical instructor or nursing staff

✦ Failure to document nursing assessments, interventions, evaluation of care

✦ Performing nursing actions without supervision when supervision is required

✦ Any nursing action or event that could result in harm or death of a client

Criteria also need to include expectations for attendance, tardiness, and professional attire. Other clinical expectations as outlined in Chapter 2 also serve as guidelines for evaluation.

USING FEEDBACK EFFECTIVELY

Feedback provides students information on their strengths and weaknesses. The more timely the feedback, the more powerful it is. Feedback helps to define for students the expectations on what they need to do each week to meet the clinical performance outcomes.

The fear of giving positive feedback in clinical is shared by many clinical instructors. Instructors are afraid that if they give positive feedback when there are still many things the student needs to do better that they will be sending the message that the student does not need to improve. LET GO OF THAT FEAR! Positive feedback is so much more powerful than negative feedback. The challenge is to isolate the action the student is doing correctly from the action they need to improve.

Negative feedback is difficult for most clinical instructors because it is hard to change negative feedback, laden with emotion, into constructive feedback that maintains the students' self-esteem. It is important that both positive and negative feedback be given in a timely manner to reinforce positive behavior and to correct the inappropriate actions before they become habits. Ongoing feedback creates a trusting partnership between the faculty and the student. If clinical instructors choose to give feedback only at midterm and the final, this creates anxiety, fosters lack of trust, and does not provide support for student learning and success.

Here are some important elements of feedback:

+ Be specific about behaviors observed

+ Describe who, what, when, where and how

+ Be timely

+ Give in private; never in front of others

+ Use "I" statements to relate your reactions

The following "Pitfalls" illustrate what NOT to do! When you were a student, you may have experienced some of these negative strategies from your clinical instructor.

+ No news is good news
  Pitfall: Students think they are doing well or they are not doing anything well

+ Negative body language like "The Look" or pointing at the student
  Pitfall: Students think you are angry but they do not know why or are afraid of you

+ The Snapback—responding immediately without thinking in a harsh tone
  Pitfall: Students become intimidated and clinical instructor looks and is out of control

+ Judgmental
  Pitfall: Destroys the student's self-esteem

Feedback is also ineffective and unacceptable when clinical instructors express themselves in highly emotional terms or make dire predictions of consequences like, "If you do not do better, you will never be a good nurse" or "You are not going to pass this clinical if you do not improve." It is Never Ever acceptable to call the student stupid or even to insinuate they are dumb or any other negative connotation. Any of the above statements will immediately destroy trust you have with the students and will result in their loss of respect for you as a clinical instructor.

Feedback often requires judgment by the clinical instructor. Here are two examples of a student failing to meet the expectation of being prepared for clinical that have two different outcomes.

EXPECTATION IS STUDENTS COME PREPARED FOR CLINICAL

Example 1:

> A student comes unprepared to clinical and states, "I was unable to find the information on my medications I am to give today."
>
> *Instructor Action*: The student should be sent home and given a clinical day failure.
>
> *Rationale*: This constitutes an unsafe care environment for the client and the student failed to meet a basic expectation for clinical.

Example 2:

> Student says, "I was unable to find the information on my drugs I am to give today. I looked in my medication book and searched the web. This morning I plan to call pharmacy to get the information on the drug."
>
> *Instructor Action*: Give positive feedback
>
> *Rationale*: The student's action represents information searching and problem solving, both excellent critical thinking attributes.

IMPLEMENTING THE EVALUATION PROCESS AND DOCUMENTATION

The concept map provides a valuable tool for you to use in teaching and evaluating the students' progress in clinical. What students write on their concept map is an external representation of their thinking. The most important aspect of the concept map is that you can see the progression of their thinking and the development of their clinical judgment. The concept map is an evolving document that changes as client conditions change and as students improve their ability to provide appropriate care and make clinical judgments. Below are some tips for using the concept map as an evaluation tool.

+ The value of requiring a concept map before clinical is to assure students are safe and are prepared for clinical.

+ It is impossible for the concept map to be 100% correct before the student has assessed the client.

+ The emphasis on evaluation and/or grading the concept map should be placed on the student's ability to make changes based on their assessment of the client, the client's response to the care, and evaluation and judgment about the care given.

The clinical instructor knows the student is becoming more sophisticated in their clinical reasoning when they are able to evaluate and use clinical judgment to make decisions about what care is needed in the future. A rubric that can be used to grade the concept map can be found at the end of this Chapter 4.

As we stated earlier, evaluation is an ongoing process. Clinical instructors are looking for trends in students' clinical performance. Weekly evaluations are essential to identify trends. Students need timely feedback, and it is not acceptable to only do a mid-term and final evaluation. The advantages of weekly evaluations are that they provide:

+ Trends: positive or negative

+ Documentation

+ Timely feedback

+ Motivate student development

+ Assist clinical instructors with clinical assignments

In order to do an evaluation, you need a tool that accurately reflects the clinical outcomes the faculty have determined are necessary for this clinical. The tool then lists the criteria necessary for the students to meet the outcomes. In other words, do your evaluation criteria measure what you want your students to achieve? A well-constructed evaluation tool can be used weekly, at mid-term and for the final evaluation (see evaluation tool included at the end of the chapter). The **Example Evaluation Tool** included at the end of the chapter reflects the nursing process, patient safety standards, clinical application of key NCLEX® standards, professional behaviors, and required written clinical care plans or concept maps. The course syllabus must state the process for clinical evaluation to include when counseling is necessary and what constitutes clinical day failures and when the clinical day failures result in course failure (see **Example of Policies for the Course Syllabus** at the end of the chapter).

Anecdotal notes are an excellent supplement to the weekly evaluation tool. They are the personal property of the clinical instructor and include information not on the weekly evaluation tool. They are not part of the permanent record unless the clinical instructor makes them available to others. Good anecdotal notes are the story behind your observations, a way to capture your thoughts, or the message your "gut" is giving you. We have all had moments in clinical with a student where the red flag went up but you just could not put your finger on it. The anecdotal notes are the place to write the objective information surrounding that event. They provide a more detailed account of the student's clinical performance that day. In addition, they can serve as excellent backup documentation when a student needs to fail clinical (see an **Example of Anecdotal Notes** at the end of the chapter).

Weekly evaluation of the student provides you the necessary information about the student's progress. This is where the trends become evident. Questions you want to ask yourself:

✦ Is the student receiving "satisfactory" every week and making acceptable progress?

✦ Is the student receiving some "needs improvement" in certain areas but you observe progress in the area the next week?

Action: None needed, continue to evaluate and document student's progress

But:

✦ Is the student receiving "needs improvement or unsatisfactory" in the same areas over a number of weeks with no progress?

Action: Counseling session needed.

Counseling serves to notify the student formally their performance is unsatisfactory. There are two levels of counseling:

✦ The counseling session identifies needed actions or behaviors to progress and includes consequences if they do not improve.

✦ The counseling session identifies a significant event or action that resulted in, or potentially could have resulted in, patient harm and the ensuing consequences, i.e., clinical day failure or course failure.

We recommend using the "STAR" format for counseling. This is a concise format, easy to use and keeps both clinical instructors and students focused on the facts of the situation (see **STAR Counseling Form** at the end of the chapter).

STAR

S = Situation: Describe the situation

T = Task: What was supposed to be accomplished, or what were the requirements, standards of practice or policies that were not met? Include standards or policies as appropriate.

A = Action: Plan for Action: What does the student need to do to improve?

Consequences: What are the consequences if corrective action is not taken? A time frame for improvement must be stated.

R = Results: Follow-up sessions: Were actions accomplished? What was the outcome?

When you decide that a counseling session is necessary, we recommend the following steps:

+ Inform the student that you are very concerned about their clinical performance, and you will notify them when the counseling session will occur. (DO NOT make hasty decisions you may regret or cannot support. Consult course coordinator).

+ Complete the STAR counseling form (be objective, stick to the facts). You may need to include observations from an earlier time with the specific incident and date that you included in your anecdotal notes.

+ Have the course coordinator or other neutral party review the counseling statement for clarity, appropriate steps and consequences prior to the session.

+ Notify the student and the witness of the scheduled counseling time.

+ Set the structure for the counseling session with the student when they arrive: purpose of the meeting, introduce the witness, and begin with the situation as written on the counseling form.

+ Be prepared to move the discussion back to the focus of the counseling session if the student wants to deviate to other topics.

+ If the student becomes too emotional, recognize the emotion, give the student time to collect their thoughts, and if needed, give them a break.

+ When you are done presenting the situation, give the student an opportunity to express their side of the story. (Note: there is a place on the form for the student to write their comments.)

+ After the student presents their side of the story, proceed as planned or if the student brings new information to the situation that may change actions or consequences, inform the student that you will reassess the new information and will reschedule another counseling session.

+ At the conclusion of the session, the student signs the form. If the student refuses to sign the form, let them know the signature only indicates they have seen the form and the session occurred. They can write in the comment section if they disagree. If the student still refuses to sign, just note that on the counseling form.

+ Other signatures include yours and the witness. Be sure it is dated and timed.

+ A copy is given to the student.

+ REMAIN CALM AT ALL TIMES!!!!!!

Two examples of completed **STAR Counseling Forms** are included at the end of the chapter.

Clinical instructors worry about an unsafe event that occurs on the last day of clinical. Does that warrant failing the student? It does not matter when an unsafe event occurs. If it was unsafe on the first day of clinical, it is unsafe on the last day of clinical. With a well-written and implemented evaluation process followed on a weekly basis, the clinical instructor would have the support needed to fail the student from clinical and/or the course depending on what constitutes failure.

Luckily these situations, although extremely distressing, happen infrequently. Most of the time, the evaluation process is positive. The students improve their skills and abilities, are motivated for future growth and best of all, they are successful in achieving the clinical outcomes.

CLINICAL EVALUATION TOOL

CLINICAL EVALUATION TOOL

Student Name:

Clinical Date:

PERFORMANCE OUTCOMES	S	NI	U	NA	S	NI	U	NA	S	NI	U	NA	S	NI	U	NA	S	NI	U	NA	S	NI	U	NA	S	NI	U	NA	S	NI	U	NA	S	NI	U	NA	S	NI	U	NA	S	NI	U	NA
Prepared for all facets of clinical day (skills, drugs, patho, etc.)																																												
Assessment																																												
Performs system-specific assessments; i.e., physiology, psychosocial, culture, spiritual																																												
Recognizes deviations from client's normal																																												
Analysis: Nursing Diag. Concepts, Outcomes																																												
Formulates appropriate nursing dx, concepts, desired outcomes using assessment																																												
Planning																																												
Identifies specific, measureable outcome criteria																																												
Develops interventions to obtain desired outcomes																																												
Implement Interventions																																												
Implement priority nursing interventions																																												
Perform nursing procedures with supervision as needed																																												
Med protocol (preparation/ administration/ documentation)																																												
Discuss appropriate principles of delegation, room assignment for specific client's needs																																												
Notifies instructor/ nurse (trends /changes in client condition, complications with meds and/or post procedure) & intervene as appropriate																																												
Evaluation																																												
Evaluation of progress toward desired outcomes																																												
Evaluate medications for desired outcomes, undesirable effects, interactions																																												

Page 1

CLINICAL EVALUATION TOOL (cont'd)

CLINICAL EVALUATION TOOL

Student Name:

Clinical Date:

PERFORMANCE OUTCOMES	S	NI	U	NA	S	NI	U	NA	S	NI	U	NA	S	NI	U	NA	S	NI	U	NA
Clinical Judgement																				
Assess if progress toward outcomes is being met; makes changes as appropriate																				
Safety/Infection Control																				
Seeks guidance when appropriate																				
Maintains client safety (fall prevention, bed position, call light, infection control, equipment, etc.)																				
Communication																				
Written communication/ charting is complete, timely and cosigned by end of shift																				
Oral Communication: uses therapeutic communication techniques																				
Non-verbal communication: Aware of importance & impact of non-verbal behavior																				
Gives concise, accurate, compete report at end of day following SBAR before leaving																				
Pt teaching concise, accurate; includes health promotion & plan for transitional care																				
Professional Behavior																				
Integrates standards of care, scope of practice & ethical practice into client care																				
Coordinates/colloborates/advocates with interdisciplinary team																				
Accepts constructive criticism																				
Maintains client / institutional confidentiality; i.e., HIPPA																				
Assertive in seeking learning experiences																				

CLINICAL EVALUATION TOOL (cont'd)

Student Name:

CLINICAL EVALUATION TOOL

Clinical Date:																																							
PERFORMANCE OUTCOMES	S	NI	U	NA	S	NI	U	NA	S	NI	U	NA	S	NI	U	NA	S	NI	U	NA	S	NI	U	NA	S	NI	U	NA	S	NI	U	NA	S	NI	U	NA	S	NI	U	NA
Respectful of all patients/personnel																																								
Reports on time to unit/conferences & utilizes spare time constructively																																								
Follows dress code																																								
Outcome Web																																								
Written /Oral Outcome web 1st page completed, with priority interventions identified based on assessment, evaluation of pt response & progress toward outcomes																																								
Paperwork turned in on time																																								
Faculty/student initials																																								

S: Satisfactory; NI: Needs Improvement; U: Unsatisfactory; NA: Not experienced

S: Clinical behavior is safe & demonstrates growth toward course competencies

NI: Clinical behavior is safe; however, performance is deficient in essential background knowledge

U: Clinical behavior is unsafe. Performance seldom demonstrates essential knowledge & growth toward competencies

NA: Clinical behavior not relevant to assigned patient

Absences: _____   Late arrivals: _____

Final Clinical Grade: _____

Faculty: _____   Date: _____

Student: _____   Date: _____

Comments:

Handout 2

EXAMPLE OF POLICIES FOR A SYLLABUS

CLINICAL PRACTICE ATTENDANCE POLICY

▲ *Students are expected to attend all clinical activities, including simulation lab and extrinsic sites.* Absences will be considered only if certified as unavoidable because of sickness or other causes, such as accident or death of immediate family member, and student provides documentation (such as doctor's excuse for illness, etc.).

▲ **Unexcused clinical absences will result in a clinical day failure for each missed clinical experience.**

▲ **Two clinical day failures will result in a course failure.** For example, unacceptable reasons for missing a clinical experience are work, travel, or social reasons.

▲ Make-up time for missed clinical nursing experiences will be **determined at the discretion of the course coordinator and availability of clinical facilities** and lab facilities.

▲ Failure to complete make up clinical may result in course failure.

▲ **A student will notify their clinical instructor verbally at least 1 hour prior to the absence and notify the course coordinator within 24 hours. Faculty may require withdrawal of any student who has missed sufficient clinical to prevent completion of clinical objectives.**

CLINICAL EXPECTATIONS

It is expected that students in a professional nursing program will be **consistently on time and prepared** for all lab and clinical assignments.

Any student reporting unprepared, no equipment, inappropriately dressed or not completing clinical preparation prior to clinical or any other non-professional behavior will:

▲ 1st offense = student will receive a warning and receive a written counseling statement

▲ 2nd offense = student will be sent home with Clinical Day Failure and receive a written counseling statement

▲ 3rd offense = student will be sent home and receive a Clinical Day Failure which will constitute a course failure.

TARDINESS POLICY:

Late arrival to clinical or post conference is not acceptable. Any student reporting to clinical or the lab late after the scheduled time (as scheduled weekly) is subject to penalties and consequences associated with professionalism and accountability.

▲ For the 1st offense = student will receive a verbal warning with a written counseling statement.

▲ For the 2nd offense = student will be sent home and receive a Clinical Day Failure with a written counseling statement.

▲ For a 3rd offense = student will be sent home and receive a Clinical Day Failure which will constitute a course failure.

EXAMPLE OF ANECDOTAL NOTES

9/2	Did not receive clinical assignment. Attempted to contact student at both contact numbers she had given. Was unable to reach her or leave a message at either number. Course coordinator aware of this and present during phone attempts.
9/7	Discussed assignment not received and inability to leave messages. Student stated she was out of town and has had phone and computer troubles. Turned in hard copy of assignment. Discussed the importance of timeliness of clinical work.
9/14	Student turned in assignment on time on 9/9, but had the previous week questions, she was unaware of the updated assignment. Discussed the need to ensure she checks for the updated assignments.
9/16	Student did not turn in assignment related to hyperbarics experience.
9/21	Student stated she was "unaware there was an assignment associated with this." She e-mailed it that evening. Counseled student regarding the late and inaccurate assignments. Explained so far her clinical performance was very good, but she needs to be organized and aware of deadlines and must meet these as assigned. I asked her to think about what she could do to improve in this manner. She stated she "has a lot going on," but would make every effort to do so. She said poor organization is a weakness of hers. Discussed this with course coordinator and was instructed to continue to document interactions and discussions.
9/28	Absent—was called the prior night and informed that she would be out because her daughter had an ear infection. Course coordinator notified.
11/9	Absent—contacted the night prior. Student stated she had a virus. (The next time we spoke, 10/12, student stated by clinical morning she had felt better, but her son then had the virus.)
11/16	Confirmed make-up day for 11/14 and asked about excuse. She stated she would get one as requested by course coordinator. She stated she was not given a deadline for this.
11/22	I contacted student via e-mail to let her know I had not received her ED extrinsic assignment. Student contacted me by phone that evening to let me know she had sent it that day after receiving my e-mail and must have forgotten to send it when she completed it last week. I then read her e-mail, see attached, and had to contact her again because the assignment was not attached to the e-mail. Student said she had printed a copy and would bring it to clinical the following day. Contacted course coordinator to discuss student's late assignments and absences for direction on how to proceed. As both assignments were pass/fail, Coordinator advised since they were turned in complete, they should be considered passing.
11/23	Student turned in hard copy of ED extrinsic.
11/24	Make-up clinical day

STAR COUNSELING FORM

Faculty Name: _____   Date of Incident: _____

Student Name: _____   Date of Session: _____

S – SITUATION: Describe the situation.

T – TASK: Requirements and/or policy performance standards that are not being met. (Standards and evaluation criteria published in course syllabus and/or in the University or College of Nursing student handbooks). State reference with page number(s) if applicable.

A – ACTIONS: to be taken to improve unsatisfactory performance.

Consequences: Consequences of not meeting performance improvement plan.

R – RESULTS: Date: (Results from action listed above actions to be taken)

DATE TO IMPROVE PERFORMANCE BY:

Faculty Signature: _____   Date: _____

Student Signature: _____   Date: _____

Observer Signature: _____   Date: _____

EXAMPLE STAR COUNSELING FORM

Faculty Name: <u>Dr. Seuss</u>   Date of Incident: <u>October 2, 2010</u>

Student Name: <u>Minnie Mouse</u>   Date of Session: <u>October 8, 2010</u>

S – SITUATION: Describe the situation:

1. Wore brown shoes to clinical. Stated it was because she had washed her shoes and they were not dry.
2. When asked where her stethoscope was as I observed her getting ready for her assessment, she reported it was in the conference room.
3. Conducted an equipment check at the end of clinical and she did not have stethoscope or watch.

T – TASK: Requirements and/or policy performance standards that are not being met. (Safety standards and evaluation criteria published in course syllabus.) State reference with page number(s).

   Reference: Course Syllabus. Page 8: Clinical Preparation & Dress Code

   Page 11: Statement of Academic Responsibility and clinical orientation

   Evaluation Criteria: Ethical behavior

A – ACTIONS: to be taken to improve unsatisfactory performance:

1. Come to clinical in appropriate clinical uniform with white shoes
2. Bring all equipment needed, stethoscope, watch, scissors, and protective eyewear
3. Answer questions honestly

Consequences: Consequences of not meeting performance improvement plan:

Failure to wear correct uniform and bring equipment to clinical will result in being sent home from clinical with a clinical day failure

Date to improve performance by: Begin immediately with next clinical day, Oct. 21, 2010

Faculty Signature: *Dr. Seuss*   Student Signature: *Minnie Mouse*

Observer Signature: _____

R - RESULTS: Date: (Results from action listed above)

1. Came appropriately dressed for clinical
2. Had equipment needed for clinical
3. No further incidents of dishonesty

FURTHER ACTION NEEDED (none, further counseling, consequences imposed):

No further action needed

Faculty Signature: *Dr. Seuss*   Student Signature: *Minnie Mouse*

Observer Signature: _____

Handout 6

EXAMPLE STAR COUNSELING WARNING FORM
UNSATISFACTORY COURSE PERFORMANCE CLINICAL DAY FAILURE

Faculty Name: _____   Student Name: _____

Date of Counseling Session: September 16, 2010   Date of Incident: September 10, 2010

S – SITUATION: Describe the situation. Course requirement not being met:

Gave Oxycodone, a narcotic, to her patient without the knowledge or supervision of the clinical faculty. (Reference: Number 6 under Medication Error Policy, page 10 of 323 Syllabus)

1. Could not answer questions about the actions of the medication. (Reference: Number 6 under Medication Error Policy, page 10 of 323 Syllabus)

2. Medication was not signed out, count was not done and no documentation of the medication was given. (Reference Number 5 under Medication Error Policy, page 10 of syllabus)

3. The patient was not assessed for level or type of pain. Patient's husband requested the pain medication for his wife. (Reference Number 5 under Medication Error Policy, page 10 of syllabus)

T – TASK: Requirements and/or policy performance standards that are not being met:

Reference: (Reference: Number 6 under Medication Error Policy, page 10 of Syllabus)

Student Medication Error Policy, page 10 of the Course Syllabus

Guidelines for clinical performance given in orientation for clinical on August 27, 2010

A – ACTIONS: to be taken to improve unsatisfactory performance:

1. All medications will be given under the supervision of your clinical faculty until you are notified otherwise.

2. Know the action and significant side effects of all medications prior to administering the medication.

3. All medications need to be correctly documented per hospital policy.

4. Failure to do so will result in a 2nd clinical day failure.

R – RESULTS: Date: Pending (Results from action listed above)

DATE TO IMPROVE PERFORMANCE BY: Immediately beginning with the next clinical day on Sept 17, 2010.

Faculty Signature: _____   Date: _____

Student Signature: _____   Date: _____

Observer Signature: _____   Date: _____

To be filed: Faculty files, Student file in Student Services

CHAPTER 8

Linking Clinical Experience to NCLEX® Success

IN THIS CHAPTER YOU WILL LEARN HOW TO:

→ Apply NCLEX® standards throughout the clinical experience

→ Adapt structures organized from the NCLEX® standards

APPLY NCLEX® STANDARDS THROUGHOUT THE CLINICAL EXPERIENCE

As a clinical instructor, you are one of the most important and powerful people in preparing the student nurse for success on the NCLEX®. Now that you have reviewed the chapters in this book from how to start teaching clinical to evaluating the clinical experience, let's move on to incorporating NCLEX® standards throughout the clinical experience.

Prior to linking clinical experience to NCLEX® success, it is important to begin with a review of some of the basic facts about the NCLEX-RN®. The purpose of the NCLEX-RN® is to ensure public protection. The exam evaluates specific competencies needed by the newly licensed, entry-level registered nurse to perform safely and effectively. The NCLEX-RN® Test Plan provides an abbreviated summary of the content and scope of the licensing examination. This plan is currently revised every three years. The Test Plan can be downloaded from the National Council State Board of Nursing's website (www.ncsbn.org). It provides a compass for preparation of the nursing student.

Unfortunately many clinical faculty report feeling overwhelmed by being held accountable for their students' success on the NCLEX®. There is a sense of urgency for faculty to teach everything to the nursing students, when in reality this creates a sense of chaos for both the student and the faculty member. Since you are reading this book and have made it back to this chapter, I am confident that you, too, may share some of these similar feelings. Please continue reading, because the good news is there are strategies to assist you in simplifying this overwhelming sense of responsibility and increasing successful outcomes for your students.

Linking these activities, as outlined in the NCLEX-RN® Test Plan, to the clinical experience is a very powerful strategy to ensure the students have an appropriate focus during their clinical experience. For example, whether the student is in medical-surgical, intensive care, obstetrics, or pediatric clinical, the clinical objectives should reflect the NCLEX® Activity Statements.

In order to prioritize these activities, we have adapted the mnemonics "**SAFETY**," "**RISK**," and "**AIDES**" to provide you and your students with structures for organizing some of the NCLEX® activities. (Refer to Handouts 1, 2, and 3 on pages 87-89.)

ADAPT STRUCTURES ORGANIZED FROM THE NCLEX® STANDARDS

Some examples of how you may adapt the mnemonic "**SAFETY**" to linking the clinical experience to NCLEX® success begins with us starting to review the various letters beginning with the **S** in "**SAFETY**", "**System-Specific Physiology**." No matter what clinical rotation the student is in, the student must be taught to begin developing an understanding of what is physiologically taking place with the client. As the student is just beginning clinical, it may be sufficient for the student to understand the reason a school-age child is experiencing frequent swallowing after a tonsillectomy is due to bleeding. After the student understands this physiological change, then the student needs to begin to understand the pathophysiology regarding the changes in the heart rate, respiratory rate, blood pressure, skin color and temperature, and urine output (if the bleeding is not evaluated and an early intervention is not implemented). This is a great opportunity for you to take advantage of the teaching moment and compare these vital sign changes to different developmental stages. This will begin to assist the student in making links and connections. As the student grows and develops throughout the curriculum, the student needs to also begin to compare and contrast the similarities/differences in the physiology/pathophysiology between adults and children.

With this teaching strategy, the following NCLEX® activities are reviewed:

> ✔ Identify pathophysiology related to an acute or chronic condition (i.e., signs and symptoms).
>
> ✔ Assess and respond to changes in vital signs.

Another example of how you can link clinical experience to NCLEX® success is for us to review the **S** in "**Safety**" and "**System-Specific Assessment**." No matter what clinical rotation the student is in, the student must be taught how to complete a fast system-specific assessment with a focus on the presenting symptoms versus a detailed one-hour head-to-toe assessment. The students must learn to think "assess" from the minute they walk into the client's room. Students do not come to clinical with this cognitive skill unless you teach it in every unit and practice it every clinical day. If the students are in the pediatric clinical rotation and the school-age child is bleeding after a tonsillectomy, then you, as the clinical instructor, have an excellent opportunity to assist them in connecting that the unique system-specific assessment is the frequent swallowing and recognize the vital sign changes for the specific child. After this has been reviewed, then compare these vital sign changes to different developmental stages and/or even an adult. You, as a clinical instructor, have another opportunity to assist the student in connecting the similarities and/or differences in both the system-specific assessments and the TRENDS with the hemodynamic changes that may occur with any client who is bleeding.

As the student grows within the curriculum, it is important for the student to review the differences between the system-specific assessments for a client who is bleeding post-op GI surgery, post cardiac catheterization, fracture, placenta previa, abruption placenta, etc. It is also important for the student to recognize the similarities between the hemodynamic changes that occur with any client who is bleeding. It goes without saying, that it is imperative to review the appropriate nursing interventions for the child who is bleeding following a tonsillectomy as well as comparing the differences/similarities in the nursing care for other clients who are bleeding for various reasons. With this process, you will have addressed four more NCLEX® activities.

✔ Perform focused assessment and re-assessment.

✔ Assess and respond to changes in vital signs.

✔ Recognize signs and symptoms of complications and intervene appropriately when providing care.

✔ Recognize trends and changes in client condition and intervene.

The students also need to develop the habit of reviewing "**System-specific labs and diagnostic procedures**" through analyzing labs and performing diagnostic tests (i.e., EKG, O_2 saturation, glucose monitoring, etc.). During each clinical experience, the students should develop the habit of reviewing labs and linking the significance of these to their client. In order to provide both you and your students with a structure for this, we have included a handout titled **Lab & Diagnostic Tests and Procedures Form** and a handout titled **Diagnostic Tests/Procedures** in Chapter 4. This process has addressed the following NCLEX® activities:

✔ Perform diagnostic testing.

✔ Evaluate the results of diagnostic testing and intervene as needed.

✔ Diagnostic Testing Assessment/Intervention.

✔ Lab values.

✔ Recognize signs and symptoms of complications and intervene appropriately when providing care.

The **A** in "SAFETY" stands for "**Analyzing priority nursing concepts.**" The nursing student needs to learn how to review and assess several nursing needs for several different clients and prioritize the care for these clients. This is an excellent opportunity for you to assist the student in understanding how to appropriately triage or prioritize nursing care. This can also be a great topic for pre/post conferences. The NCLEX® activity addressed for this process is:

✔ Assess/triage clients to prioritize order of care delivery.

The **F** in "SAFETY" represents what nursing interventions should be implemented "**First**" as well as what medications should be administered first. When the client has 4 nursing interventions that need implemented, then you can assist the student by consistently asking questions such as, *"What are the priority nursing actions?" "What medications should be administered first for specific clinical assessments?"* For example, if a client begins spitting out blood and the client is positioned in the supine position, then the first nursing action would be to reposition client even prior to notifying health care provider or initiating a complete assessment.

Another example of how you can assist the student in prioritizing, is if the client has respiratory problems and has an order to administer a corticosteroid inhaler and a Beta$_2$ Adrenergic Agonist such as Albuterol, then you may want to help the student in connecting the actions for both of these drugs with the pathophysiology. This will assist them in understanding the rationale for administering Albuterol prior to the steroid inhaler. This will assist in reviewing the NCLEX® activity:

✔ Prioritize workload to manage time effectively.

The **E** in "SAFETY" will assist the student in always remembering to evaluate the "**Expected Outcomes**" from the nursing care as well as from the medications.

✦ Did the bleeding stop?

✦ Did the breath sounds improve?

✦ Did the vital signs return to baseline?

✦ Did the medication assist in reducing the intracranial pressure?

✦ Did the medication assist in reducing the serum glucose?

The NCLEX® activities addressed include:

✔ Evaluate/document response to treatment.

✔ Evaluate therapeutic effect of medications.

"**Trends**" in the client's assessment, **T** in "SAFETY," is an excellent observation to determine if the client is stable. If client is not stable, then assist the students in prioritizing which nursing interventions need to be implemented immediately to prevent the client from experiencing a crisis. For example, if the client begins hemorrhaging two hours post-op, the student needs to assess the subtle changes with the heart rate and restlessness, and recognize the potential complication with bleeding prior to the client progressing to hypovolemic shock and intervene appropriately.

Another example of trends would be if the client was receiving Magnesium Sulfate and the urine output had been 85 cc/hour, and the next hour the urine output is 45 cc/hour. The Magnesium Sulfate is excreted in the urine, and with this trend it would be imperative to report this decline and not wait for the urine to continue to decline. The student needs your assistance and support to learn how to think like this. With role-modeling your thinking, this will help the student to begin understanding this process. This will take a lot of practice, but with your consistent encouragement and assistance, it will become part of the structure for thinking as the student develops and implements the plan of care. This represents a new NCLEX® activity and requires thinking at the analysis level. The NCLEX® activities reviewed include:

- ✔ Recognize trends and changes in client condition and intervene.
- ✔ Recognize signs and symptoms of complications and intervene appropriately when providing care.
- ✔ Assess and respond to changes in vital signs.

The **Y** in "SAFETY" represents management. "**Yes, Management is important to prevent "RISK" to our clients!**" Refer to Handout 2 on page 88 for examples of NCLEX® activities reflecting Management and Safety on the NCLEX®. These activities will be useful for you to connect throughout clinical for both the client safety as well as to assist with NCLEX® success. From day one in clinical, the student needs to assess the following:

- ✦ Risk for falls
- ✦ Practice infection control
- ✦ Identify client correctly
- ✦ Review accuracy of orders
- ✦ Assess and prevent skin breakdown
- ✦ Practice equipment safety
- ✦ Understand Standards of Practice
- ✦ Practice effective documentation
- ✦ Client teaching

The mnemonic "AIDES" is also a structure for organizing the NCLEX® activities that have a focus on pharmacology. This is a great tool to use throughout the curriculum, so the students in clinical know what the expectations are from semester to semester. In many situations, the clinical instructors focus on different aspects of pharmacology, and as soon as the students understand what the faculty wants, it is time for a new clinical rotation. "AIDES" reflect NCLEX® standards, so if these are consistently reviewed based on the student's educational development and position within the curriculum, students will have a great understanding of what it takes to be successful on the NCLEX®.

These three mnemonics (pages 87-89) will serve as a compass to you as well as your students while integrating NCLEX® standards during the clinical experience. Please note that while many of the NCLEX® activities from the NCLEX® Test Plan are represented throughout the mnemonics, these are not all inclusive. A complete list of these can be downloaded from the National Council of State Boards of Nursing (www.ncbn.org). It would be very powerful if we started from Day 1 in clinical adapting many of these standards and leveled these throughout the curriculum. If each clinical faculty would adapt these throughout each clinical rotation and be consistent with expectations, paperwork, and questions throughout the curriculum, nursing students would have an excellent roadmap to being successful on the NCLEX® while they are still in school. These standards can and should be the framework for the various teaching strategies outlined in previous chapters. **The Quick Approach: Inquiry Questions for Clinical Knowledge Organized Around the Nursing Process** (Chapter 3) and the **Clinical Evaluation Tool** (Chapter 7) help link clinical to NCLEX®.

Clinical nursing faculty hold a very powerful key to students' success. It is in the clinical experience where students report they begin making connections from theory to clinical practice. Linking NCLEX® with your clinical teaching and evaluating is indeed the ticket to your students' success.

SAFETY

This structure can help prioritize NCLEX® activities that can be evaluated through the **Outcome Concept Map, History and Pathophysiology Information and Reflection Questions** (see Chapter 4 handouts).

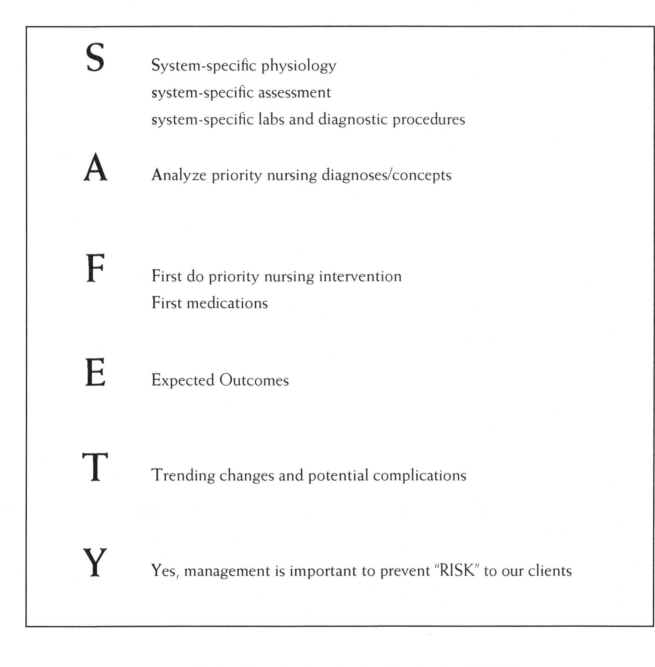

S   System-specific physiology

system-specific assessment

system-specific labs and diagnostic procedures

A   Analyze priority nursing diagnoses/concepts

F   First do priority nursing intervention

First medications

E   Expected Outcomes

T   Trending changes and potential complications

Y   Yes, management is important to prevent "RISK" to our clients

Reference: National Council of State Boards of Nursing, Inc. (NCSBN) 2009

Handout 2

RISK

A structure for prioritizing Management and Safety NCLEX® Activities. Directions: *Please complete on your patient assignment. Turn into clinical instructor* _____.

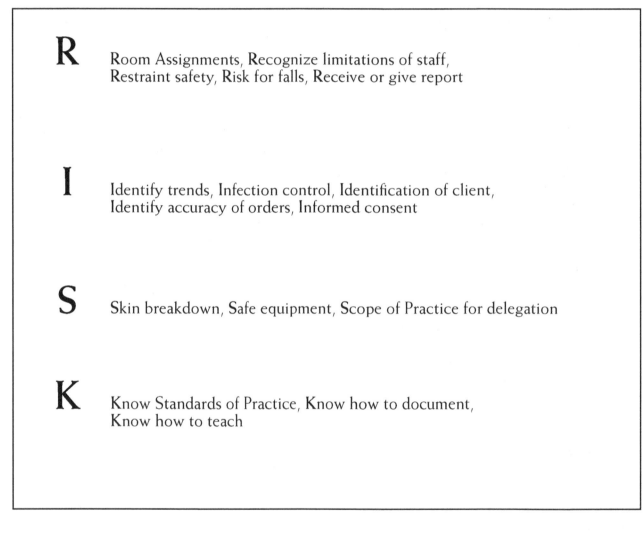

R   Room Assignments, Recognize limitations of staff, Restraint safety, Risk for falls, Receive or give report

I   Identify trends, Infection control, Identification of client, Identify accuracy of orders, Informed consent

S   Skin breakdown, Safe equipment, Scope of Practice for delegation

K   Know Standards of Practice, Know how to document, Know how to teach

Reference: National Council of State Boards of Nursing, Inc. (NCSBN) ***2009***

AIDES

A structure for prioritizing Pharmacology NCLEX® Activities. Directions: *Please complete on ___ of your priority medications. Turn into clinical instructor* _____.

NAME OF DRUG: BRAND _____   GENERIC _____

CLASSIFICATION: _____

A   Action of medication:

Administration of medication. Dosage ordered_____

How to administer:

Assessment:

Adverse Effects. List significant ones:

Accuracy/Appropriateness of order. Is it indicated based on client's condition, known allergies, drug-drug or drug-food interactions? If not, what action did you take?

I   Interactions (Drug-Drug, Food-Drug):

Identify priority plan prior to giving drug (i.e., vital signs, labs, allergies, etc.):

Identify priority plan after giving drug:

D   Desired outcomes of the drug:

Discharge teaching—Administration considerations for client and family:

E   Evaluate signs and symptoms of complications. Intervene if necessary and describe:

S   Safety (client identification, risk for falls, vital sign assessments):

Reference: National Council of State Boards of Nursing, Inc. (NCSBN) 2009

NOTES

Bibliography

Asby, F.G. & Maddox, W.T. (2010). Human category learning 2.0., Annals NY Academy Science, December 2010.

Benner, P., Sutphen, M., Leonard, V., & Day, L. (2010). Educating nurses: A call for radical transformation. San Francisco: Jossey-Bass.

Benner, P., Tanner, C., & Chesla, C. (2008). Expertise in nursing practice. New York, NY: Springer Publishing Company, LLC.

Clark, C. (2008). Student perspectives on faculty incivility in nursing education: An application of the concept of rankism. *Nursing Outlook, 56*, 4-8.

Creech, C. (2008). Are we moving toward an expanded role for part-time faculty? *Nurse Educator, 33*, 31-34.

Dolan, G. (2003). Assessing student nurse clinical competency: Will we ever get it right? *Journal of Clinical Nursing, 12*, 132-141.

Gaberson, K.B. & Oermann, M.H. (2006). Clinical teaching strategies for nursing. New York, NY: Springer Publishing Company.

Herman, J.W. (2008). Creative teaching strategies for the nurse educator. Philadelphia, PA: F.A. Davis.

Holden, C. (2009). Multitasking muddles the mind? http://news.sciencemag.org/sciencenow/2009/08/25-02.html. Retrieved 12-1-2010.

Luhanga, F., Yonge, O.J., & Myrick, R. (2008). Failure to assign failing grades. *International Journal of Nursing Education Scholarship, 5*, 1-14.

Manning, L. & Rayfield, S. (2009). Pharmacology made insanely easy. Duluth, GA: I CAN Publishing®, Inc.

National Council of State Boards of Nursing. (2009). Report of findings from the 2008 RN practice analysis: Linking the NCLEX-RN® examination to practice. Chicago, IL.

Penn, B.K. (Ed.). (2008). Mastering the teaching role: A guide for nurse educators. Philadelphia, PA: F.A. Davis.

Pesut, D. & Herman, J.A. (1999). Clinical reasoning: The art and science of critical and creative thinking. Albany, NY: Delmar Publishing.

Rayfield, S. & Manning, L. (2009). Pathways of teaching nursing: Keeping it real! Duluth, GA: I CAN Publishing®, Inc.

Rayfield, S. & Manning, L. (2010). NCLEX-RN® 101: How to pass! Duluth, GA: I CAN Publishing®, Inc.

Skiba, D. & Barton, A. (2006). Adapting your teaching to accommodate the NET generation of learners. *The Online Journal of Issues in Nursing.* 11(2), Manuscript 4. Available: http://www.nursingworld.org/MainMenuCategories/ANAMarketplace/ANAPeriodicals/OJIN/Table of Contents/Volume112006/No2May06/tpc30_416076.aspx. Retrieved 12-15-2010.

Tanner, C. (2006). Thinking like a nurse: A research-based model of clinical judgment in Nursing. *Journal of Nursing Education*, 45, 204-211.

Zbat-Kan, E. & Stabler-Haas, S. (2009). Fast facts for the clinical nursing instructor: Clinical teaching in a nutshell. New York, NY: Springer Publishing Company.

Index

Other Books Published by I CAN Publishing®, Inc.

NCLEX-RN® 101: How to Pass!

NCLEX-PN® 101: How to Pass!

Nursing Made Insanely Easy!

Pharmacology Made Insanely Easy!

Pathways of Teaching Nursing: Keeping it Real!

★ ★ ★ ★ ★ ★ ★ ★ ★ ★ ★ ★ ★ ★ ★ ★ ★ ★ ★

CDs for Educators

Nursing Made Insanely Easy! Images on CD

Pharmacology Made Insanely Easy! CD review

★ ★ ★ ★ ★ ★ ★ ★ ★ ★ ★ ★ ★ ★ ★ ★ ★ ★ ★

I CAN Publishing®, Inc.
2650 Chattahoochee Drive, Suite 100
Duluth, GA 30097
866.428.5589
www.icanpublishing.com

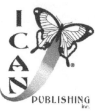